Beth,

Be well!

Hitting the Wall

Memoir of a Cancer Journey

Barbara Pate Glacel

To the sick,

While there is life there is hope.

—Cicero

Published by
Hara Publishing
P.O. Box 19732
Seattle, WA 98109
(425) 775-7868

ISBN: 1-883697-73-5
LOC: 2001089615

Manufactured in the United States
10 9 8 7 6 5 4 3 2

Editor: Vicki McCown
Desktop Publishing: Scott Carnz

This book is dedicated to

Jennifer, Sarah, and Ashley,
who saw me through the fire,
and in hopes
that a cure will be found
before they risk the flames

and to

Toni, Mary Jane, and Carolyn,
who lived and died
with dignity and grace and
provided inspiration for all survivors

Contents

Acknowledgments

Storytelling is never a solitary activity. Others are the characters, listeners, supporters, and facilitators, all of whom make the final story better than it could have been without them.

At the risk of leaving someone out, there are many people whom I must thank. First, my heartfelt thanks to the medical professionals who guided my journey and held me through the treatment, specifically Dr. Chris Georgantopoulos, Dr. Dina Hertens, Dr. Lou Diehl, Dr. Dave Jacques, Dr. Frank Ward, Dr. Ken Block, Dr. Jim Hines, Dr. Charles Day, Dr. Michael Grant, Dr. Paul West, Dr. Clorinda Zawacki, Dr. Carole Ortenzo, oncology nurse Jane Shotkin, nurse Angela Shields, physical therapists Marie Joris, Peno Carter, and Linda Pace.

Thanks and huge hugs to my e-mail support group that grew to over 100 family, friends, business colleagues, and cancer survivors, some of whom I never met. Thanks to the funny-story group of cancer patients, Howard, Andy, and Christine, all of us helping one another through a difficult time. Special thanks to Rhonda Curry, who started me on the path of learning about my disease and finding hope that I could survive.

Thanks to Bea Sadowsky who inspired me with her survivorship. Becky Hoag saw me through the hard time of hospitalization and chemo, providing meals, clothes, love, and cheer. Linda Cox became my guardian angel in so many ways, both in the United States and from afar. Shannon Wall and I shared our journeys, helping one another to sort out meaning. Thanks and prayers for the ladies of the breast cancer support groups of Mons, Belgium, and Killeen, Texas.

Several people were instrumental in guiding my journey through breast cancer. My mother, Virginia Pate Wetter, has always been my role model for how to confront adversity with grace. My sister, Dr. Kennon Pate McKee, was always there for me, helping to keep me positive, to analyze my feelings, and to share my pain.

My family, of course, deserves the greatest praise. My husband, Bob, was with me through every inch of the cancer journey. He also supported my need to go away by myself to tell this story. I could not have survived without him. Our daughters, Jennifer, Sarah, and Ashley, each helped me in her own way. Jenn shared the receipt of the devastating diagnosis and mothered me through surgery. Sarah gave wise counsel on how I could go on as a whole person. Ashley massaged my bald head and joined me in healing laughter.

Several people read the manuscript and offered good suggestions and corrections on medical information. Thanks to Dr. Robert Wascher, nurse Diana Ruzicka, breast cancer advocate Rosemary Locke, authors Diane Cole and Musa Mayer, and my sister, Kennon. Finding a publisher was no small feat. My gratitude for assistance on this search goes to Elaine Biech, Dan Smetanka, Ed Helvey, Jack Covert, and Kathy Welton. My publisher, Sheryn Hara, and editor, Vicki McCown, offered valuable suggestions to improve the manuscript and deliver it to readers.

Finally, I salute the courage of the many women and men who suffer with the terrible disease of breast cancer. It is my fervent hope that my story will help those who must travel the road of cancer diagnosis and treatment.

Preface

This story of cancer, support, hope, and life has been two years in the living and the writing. The story has lived inside me, wanting desperately to come out. It is made up of many journal writings and a selection of the hundreds and hundreds of messages to and from friends over this period of time. The compilation of all these thoughts has been a cathartic exercise for me and, I hope, will be helpful to others who go through the incredible experience of cancer. It is truly a life-changing event both for the patient and for those who wage the battle alongside the patient.

When I was diagnosed with breast cancer in December 1996, my world stopped. It felt as though I had hit a wall while racing at breakneck speed. My total focus changed from everyday life to learning more about the disease, the options, and the healing. Over time, my healing demanded that I let the story come out of me and be put to paper. I needed to go someplace where I would be completely focused on the experience and my spirit would be nourished. I chose Williamsburg, a place familiar to me since childhood, where three generations of my family have attended The College of William and Mary, and where I have many happy memories.

Bob and I own a home in Williamsburg where we spend too little time. I came alone and set up my writing room in the dining room. It is a lovely place to write. The dining room overlooks the forested back of the house with a huge bay window in front of me viewing trees across the road. The many birds, the bright sunshine, the quiet setting combine to make it a peaceful and bright place to be creative.

I am surrounded by the reams of printed-out e-mail messages from the past two years, many books, letters, get-well cards and memorabilia, and all the photos and symbols of the time during my treatment that serve as a stimulus to remember and to write. Pictures of my husband, Bob, and our daughters, Jenn, Sarah, and Ashley, sit next to my computer as they sat on my night table in the Jules Bordet hospital in Belgium. The little red-hatted gnome, the cross that reads *Je suis avec vous*, the silver shaman pin, the chakra worry beads, the bag of turquoise, the Race for the Cure survivor pin, the luminary with my name on it from the Relay for Life, my birthday brooch, and the rose-gold breast cancer ribbon—all these symbols and mementos are vivid reminders.

Just this week, as I have been writing, I have learned of another friend diagnosed with breast cancer. The news brings back vivid memories of my own diagnosis. It is truly so frightening to get the news that one has a malignancy. What an ugly word. Only through our tireless efforts to help one another and to support research will we conquer this dreaded disease that will strike over 182,000 women in the United States in this year alone.

Today, the day that my story finished its transfer to paper, is Valentine's Day. Bob sent me a dozen red roses with a note saying he missed me. In front of me sits the valentine that he sent two years ago just as I started chemotherapy. I still had hair, but only one breast and a new scar across my chest. The words on that card are even more appropriate today:

> *For the One I Love,*
> *After so many years of picking out valentines for you, I feel like I've already said "I love you" in every way possible. But I don't know if I've put into words how grateful I am that we've come through so much together or how sharing my life with you means even more to me as time goes by. I only hope you know that after so many years, I love you in so many ways. Happy Valentine's Day.*
> *I love you,*
> *Bob*

When I finished writing this story, I had an amazing reaction. I cried. The story that had vividly lived inside was now out. I called Bob and thanked him for the tremendous support and love he has given me throughout this journey. It is true that life is now richer, the highs are higher, and the lows are manageable with love.

Williamsburg, Virginia, February 14, 1999

Characters

Many friends and family accompanied me on this cancer journey. Those who are mentioned throughout the memoir are listed below in alphabetical order by first name unless only the last name was used in the memoir.

Andy and Lynne are long-time Army friends who live in Virginia. Andy was diagnosed and treated for prostate cancer and joined the funny story group of cancer patients.

Ashley is my youngest daughter and lived at home during my cancer treatment.

Bea is the first woman I knew to have breast cancer. From my hometown, she has been a family friend for most of my life and provided support and inspiration during my treatment.

Becky and Randy are Army friends who live in Brussels. Becky cared for me from the time of hospitalization through chemotherapy.

Bob is my husband. At the time of my treatment, he was a brigadier general assigned to the Supreme Headquarters, Allied Powers Europe (SHAPE), the military arm of NATO.

Bodil is my Norwegian "sister." As an exchange student in 1966, I lived with her family in Oslo and we have remained friends for thirty-five years. She currently lives in Stockholm, Sweden.

Dr. Chris Georgantopoulos is a Canadian doctor who cared for me throughout my cancer journey.

Christine is an American woman married to a diplomat from Netherlands, living in Brussels. She had a recurrence of breast cancer, which metastasized to her liver, and she was a member of the funny story group.

Colin is my nephew, son of Howard and Kennon. He spent a year in France during the time of my treatment.

Dr. Dave Jacques was the chief of surgery, Walter Reed Army Medical Center. He advised me by phone from the day of my diagnosis.

Dr. Dina Hertens is the Belgian surgeon who performed both cancer operations at the Jules Bordet Cancer Institute.

Ethel Soriano is a holistic healer and friend of my sister Kennon. She has studied with native healers in Central and South America.

Howard is married to my sister Kennon. He was treated for colon cancer and was a member of the funny story group.

Jane Shotkin is an oncology nurse at Walter Reed Army Medical Center who advised me by phone about the side effects of chemotherapy.

Janine and Paul are Belgian friends who helped me navigate the Belgian medical system.

Jenn is my eldest daughter, a student at the College of William and Mary during my treatment.

Dr. Jim Hines was a retired doctor and friend of Kennon in Chicago. He advised me on chemotherapy and said a good doctor should "hold" the patient throughout treatment.

Jim Lewis is my cousin, an Episcopal priest who performed Bob's and my wedding ceremony. His wife, Judy, is a breast cancer survivor and oncology nurse.

Keiju is our Finnish exchange "daughter" who lived in our home for one year and went on to medical school in Finland.

Kennon is my older sister. She is a Jungian analyst and clinical psychologist in Chicago. She and my brother-in-law, Howard, are parents to Colin.

Dr. Kenton is a fictitious name for the oncologist who treated me at the Jules Bordet Cancer Institute in Brussels.

Linda is a long-time friend and godmother to our daughter Sarah. Linda accompanied me on a trip to Williamsburg during my chemotherapy, and I dubbed her my guardian angel.

Dr. Lou Diehl was chief of oncology at the Walter Reed Army Medical Center. He consulted with me by phone and followed up on my treatment on our return from Belgium.

Madame Carstairs is the *Vivre Comme Avant* volunteer who visited me in the hospital.

Marie is the physical therapist at the Mons Medical Clinic who treated my affected arm after surgery and helped me navigate the Belgian medical system.

Marilyn is a friend with multiple sclerosis who serves as a role model for courage and perseverance.

Mary Jane was a friend who had a recurrence of breast cancer and was treated with a stem cell transplant in Texas. She participated in the Relays for Life, but ultimately lost her battle to cancer.

Max was my friend and professional mentor who died of leukemia. His courage was an inspiration to me.

Mieke is a friend who lived in Brussels. She introduced me to Christine and provided support during my treatment.

Nancy is an American Navy wife who lived in Mons and provided tremendous support throughout my treatment.

Paddy is an American who began the Mons breast cancer support group.

Dr. Pincher is a fictitious name for the chief of oncology at the Jules Bordet Cancer Institute who refused to treat me.

Rhonda is my college sorority sister and a breast cancer survivor. She is the first person I called to ask for advice after my diagnosis.

Sarah is my second daughter. During the time of my treatment, she lived in Lomonosov, Russia, as an exchange student.

Shannon is a professional colleague who was diagnosed with breast cancer as I finished chemotherapy. We helped each other explore the spiritual side of our treatment.

Toni was an Army wife diagnosed with breast cancer in Texas. After three years of extensive treatment, she lost her battle.

Part One
Cancer

Getting your breast cut off

will not make things go back to normal;

your life has been changed,

and it will never be the same again.

—*Dr. Susan M. Love, M.D.*

Diagnosis—Hitting the Wall

Breast cancer had never been a huge concern to me. No one in my family had breast cancer. I had regular mammograms with negative results. Generally, I enjoyed very good health. Simply not a problem. My mother had a benign lump removed some years before as did our daughters' caregiver, Mrs. Fox. I actually didn't even know very many people who had breast cancer, or at least didn't know them well. When I was about seventeen, my mother's friend Bea had breast cancer. She had been a good friend to us after my father's death when I was just eleven. Her four daughters were friends of mine, and I remember when she was diagnosed and treated.

My college sorority sister, Rhonda, had also had breast cancer. We had remained close friends over the years, but I didn't see her often and I did not remember many of the details of her case. Being married to a career Army officer, I was often living somewhere remote when the news about others' health problems surfaced. I really was quite ignorant about breast cancer and its causes, treatment, and prognosis.

So, when I had an annual physical in November 1996, I did not question the doctor who told me that I did not need a mammogram. Since age forty I had had annual mammograms and my last mammogram had been fifteen months earlier. But the military doctor at the U.S. health clinic in Germany explained that there was a new philosophy. Women between forty and fifty years of age would have a mammogram only every two years. He performed a manual breast exam and that was that.

He did, however, put me on a mild diuretic for slightly elevated blood pressure. Since February of that year, I had been running a blood pressure

3

considered marginally high. Because my father had died at the age of forty-four of cardiac and circulatory problems, that worried me. I had explained my family history to the doctor giving me the physical. As we discussed my blood pressure, he gave an unconcerned response about the marginality of the numbers.

However, about ten minutes later, he asked, "Your parents, both alive and well?"

I wanted to sarcastically reply, "My father is as dead as he was a few minutes ago when I told you my family history." However, I more politely reminded him, "No, as I told you a few minutes ago, my father died at the age of forty-four of heart-related problems."

The doctor nearly jumped out of his chair. "Oh my goodness," he exclaimed, "Of course you must go on blood pressure medication!" Perhaps I should have known then that he was not paying much attention to my personal medical situation.

He was not my regular doctor, but a family practice physician at the U.S. Air Force Executive Health Clinic in Germany. Bob and I lived in Mons, Belgium, where he was the Director of Policy and Programmes for the Supreme Headquarters, Allied Powers Europe (SHAPE), the military arm of NATO. Bob loved the job. It allowed him frequent travel to all the NATO capitals around Europe, and provided us with a social group representing the sixteen NATO nations. Our medical care at SHAPE, however, consisted of only a small health clinic with specialized care provided in the local Belgian hospitals or in U.S. facilities in Germany. As an Army brigadier general, Bob used the Executive Services clinic in Germany, a three-hour drive away, for our annual physicals. For routine care, we depended on our small clinic.

On our return to SHAPE, I found a physician who would follow me as I began taking the blood pressure medication. A dedicated and overworked Greek-Canadian Air Force officer who had done his residency in cardiology, Dr. Christopher Georgantopoulos opened his office on a Saturday morning in order to fit me in right away as I began taking the diuretic. He gave me a modified physical and looked over the earlier results.

"Why," he asked, "didn't you have an annual mammogram this year?"

I explained that the doctor had animatedly described to me the recent conference he had attended where two Harvard physicians screamed at each other from the podium about their different philosophies on mammography. One supported annual mammograms for women over the age of forty, the other insisting that was overkill.

"Maybe so," Dr. Georgantopoulos replied, "but your history is different. You definitely need an annual mammogram."

In 1988, eight years earlier, I had begun natural menopause at age thirty-nine. My experience at that time should have convinced me not to believe blindly in doctors. I visited at least half a dozen doctors, both men and women, who told me a variety of things and sometimes irresponsibly prescribed medications. Granted, it is rare to start menopause at thirty-nine, but approximately 5 percent of American women do.

A well-regarded and expensive gynecologist in Georgetown told me simply, "Oh, you're close to forty and strange things happen to your body. Go home."

A female gynecologist in her sixties said, "Maybe you're menopausal. Take these hormones and you'll stop having hot flashes. Come back if you have a problem."

Having read the pros and cons of hormone replacement therapy (HRT), I did not want that answer either. I finally went to the hometown gynecologist who had treated me years before when I lost a pregnancy during a family visit. He had been so kind in dealing with the miscarriage, and I trusted his small-town, personal approach to medicine. For some years after that, I programmed my gynecological needs around my visits back to see my mother.

My hometown doctor took me off the hormones, ran tests, and determined that I had indeed gone through early menopause. We then tested and determined the best hormone treatment and levels for my own body and comfort. We talked long and hard about the pros and cons, but we agreed that, in my case, the advantages outweighed the disadvantages. I had a history of heart disease in my family and HRT helps the heart. I had all the risk factors except one—smoking—for osteoporosis, and my grandmother had severe osteoporosis. HRT decreases calcium loss. Also, I was having debilitating hot flashes.

I remember when my mother-in-law went through menopause. I couldn't figure out why she complained about something as silly as feeling warm. Suddenly, I understood and felt remorse at my earlier lack of sympathy. I had hot flashes so severe that they left me wringing wet. My silk blouses and business suits became pretty rumpled, and it was hard to look professional for a whole day. At night, I slept with a large towel next to the bed so I could dry off several times during the night. To me, the hormones were a gift from heaven, making me comfortable again.

Given my eight years on HRT and hearing that the family practice physician had not ordered a mammogram, Dr. Georgantopoulos was appalled. Considering that breast cancer is estrogen-dependent, he explained, my age was of less importance than the fact that I had been on HRT for so long. He ordered an immediate mammogram.

Medical care for an American in Belgium is a cultural experience. My French is moderate, but it is still a challenge to get medical care in a second language. When I checked in at the Hornu Institute of Medical Specialists, I received a whole sheet of printed labels with my name and pertinent information. I took the labels to another desk where I checked in for my mammography appointment. Soon, a man called, "Madame Glacel."

He took me to a small dressing room and instructed me to remove everything from the waist up and then come into the next room. I asked him about a drape, and he looked very surprised. Of course, he did not have a drape. Simply remove my clothing and come find him. Welcome to Belgian modesty—or lack of same. I complied with his request and removed my blouse and bra, then entered the mammography room. At least I knew what to expect here, having had half a dozen mammograms during the last eight years.

The technician did the requisite positioning, squashing, and picture-taking, and then asked me to wait again in the dressing room. They would call me in a moment for a breast ultrasound. I had never had an ultrasound of my breast, but such a procedure was routine in Belgium. I began to shiver as I waited in the dressing room, so I draped my blouse around me. I seemed to wait quite a long time, and I wondered if anyone knew I was there or whether they had forgotten me. I did not want to get dressed to go find out, and then have to get undressed again.

Eventually, the technician summoned me and took me to a different room. Uncovered from the waist up, I lay on a table and saw a doctor working with his back to me. As I waited, numerous people, mostly men, wandered in and out of the room. It seemed quite bizarre that this half-naked woman (me) lay on a table in what looked to be a thoroughfare, but it did not seem to faze them at all. Finally, I closed my eyes. An old joke came to mind about the little boy running through the girls' locker room, shouting, "Close your eyes, girls, I'm coming through." Like the girls in the locker room, if I did not see the pedestrian traffic, maybe they wouldn't see me.

Finally, the doctor stopped his work and turned to me. He spoke a little English, and he explained the ultrasound procedure. He scanned both breasts, but returned often to the outside of the right breast. He showed me on the screen a dark area on the outside and a shadow on the inside. He said they would do a *ponctionne*. I had no clue what that meant.

"Can you do that at Hornu?" I asked.

"Oh, yes," he replied. "We'll do it right now. It won't hurt."

Once again, I should have known better. Twenty-five years earlier, a male doctor told me the same thing when he did a uterine biopsy. "It won't hurt," he assured me. "You don't have much feeling in your uterus." Seconds later, as he peeled me off the ceiling, I gasped, "How do you know what it feels like since you don't have a uterus?"

The *ponctionne* was actually a needle aspiration. The doctor sprayed something unknown on my skin (probably lidocaine), located the spot on the outside of my breast by using the ultrasound to find the dark area, and inserted a huge needle. He then moved it around inside the tissue in order to aspirate some fluid. It wasn't as bad as childbirth, but I knew he had never had it done to himself, so what did he know about hurting? Nonetheless, I behaved myself. He told me I could get dressed and my Canadian doctor would receive the results in three or four days.

Bob had gone out of town for a week, and I did not want to bother him about a questionable mammogram. They were being conservative, I thought, and I agreed with that approach. Still, I felt anxious. We have three daughters, and I thought just briefly about the implications for them. I did not want to alarm them either. Jenn was in the States, a junior at the College of William and Mary, in the midst of exams. Sarah was spending a year in Russia as an exchange student, feeling pretty homesick as Christmas approached. Ashley, the only daughter still at home, didn't need to be worried.

Just the week before, my brother-in-law, Howard, had been diagnosed with colon cancer. My sister and I had talked about the anxiety of waiting for the diagnosis and about the ugly word "malignancy." When Howard's wait for results ended, the news was not good. Not only were we very upset about his health, the diagnosis put a damper on our Christmas plans. Howard and my sister, Kennon, had planned a trip to Belgium for Christmas. Their son, Colin, spending a year in France between high school and college, had arranged to come meet them. We had been excited about a wonderful family Christmas together. But Howard's diagnosis canceled their trip. Our Christmas looked to be small and bleak, without Sarah coming from Russia, either.

As darkness arrived early each day, I found myself feeling pretty down. An interminable three-day wait created uncertainty and more fear. When I received no news, I called Chris Georgantopoulos. Unable to reach him, I asked the head nurse at the clinic to call Hornu. She learned that they were still studying the fluid.

To calm my nerves, she said, "It is good news that nothing definitive has shown up. They'll call us the beginning of next week."

When Bob returned from his business trip on Saturday, I gave him the news. He seemed stoic, as always, and sure everything would be all right. On Sunday, my nerves got the better of me. I don't even remember what the issue was, but Ashley and I were arguing about something, and I dissolved into tears.

In a rare emotional outburst, I exclaimed, "I cannot always do what everyone else wants! Why don't you consider what I want sometimes, too?"

Scheduled to call Sarah that night in Russia, I felt too unsettled to make the call and be my usual cheery self. Bob placed the call by himself, and before I knew what he was doing, he told Sarah about the mammogram. I raced into the room.

"Don't tell her that!" I admonished, thankful that Ashley had not heard. Obviously, any bad news worried Sarah while she lived so far from home.

Bob held out the phone to me, and after a moment's hesitation, I took it.

"It's nothing," I told her. "I'm tired and sad that you and Aunt Kennon's family won't be here for Christmas. That's all. I'll send you an e-mail at your friend's house if there's any problem with the tests."

On Monday, Chris Georgantopoulos called. Hornu wanted to do a tissue biopsy because the fluid biopsy was inconclusive. Not to worry, this was simply standard procedure. Could I go back to Hornu the next day? Of course. I didn't know what was involved with the tissue biopsy, but I knew I didn't want to go alone. I called Bob at the office and asked if he could take me the next day. I sent Sarah a vague e-mail message, saying that the results were fine and I would have more tests later. I didn't want to lie, but I didn't want her to be worried either.

By now, I knew the procedure at Hornu. Get the labels, check in at mammography, wait to be called. Go in the dressing room, take off everything from waist up, come to the mammography room where four people were waiting for me. But I was not prepared for the procedure. The technician placed a stool in front of the mammography machine and adjusted the height of the machine to my right breast. For about thirty minutes, she positioned, squashed, took pictures, drew on my breast, and repositioned to start over. Finally, the suspicious area was correctly identified and labeled. With my breast still inserted in the mammography machine, a series of needles were injected to pull out more fluid and, finally, tissue.

Periodically, especially when I stopped breathing, someone would look at me and say, "*Ca va?*" which is to say, "Everything ok?" It actually hurt like the dickens, but I breathed deeply and nodded. Finally, they were finished. Everyone was very kind and concerned, and I appreciated their treatment.

Waiting for news again seemed torturous, but life went on with work and Ashley's activities. Jenn arrived home at the end of the week for the Christmas holidays. She napped in the afternoon, having flown all night from the States. As I wrapped last-minute gifts, the phone rang.

It was Chris Georgantopoulos. "I have the report from Hornu. Do you want to come in to talk about the results?" he asked. That was a dead give away.

"No," I responded, "you can tell me on the phone."

Gently, Chris explained that he had bad news. His translation of the French lab report indicated that I had invasive ductal cancer with one confirmed site and one suspicious site. The pathologist recommended an immediate mastectomy.

"What do we do now?" I asked, but barely heard his answer.

Timing created a problem with Christmas and holidays for the next ten days. However, Chris would try to get the earliest possible appointment at the Jules Bordet Cancer Institute in Brussels. Bordet is a world-class teaching hospital dedicated to the treatment of cancer, and Chris felt confident this was where I would want to be treated in Belgium.

"Do you want a prescription to help you sleep?" he asked.

"No, thanks, Chris. Have a good weekend."

Hearing my wooden tone, he gave me his home phone number in the event I wanted him over the weekend. We agreed to talk on Monday.

With Jenn still asleep, I called Bob at the office. Luckily, he answered on his private line. I could not have spoken to anyone else.

I said simply, "Chris called. I think you'd better come home."

"What's the report?" he asked.

"It's about as bad as it could possibly be," I responded, and then I started crying.

I waited for Bob to arrive, lost in a daze. I could not remember what Chris had said. Jenn only awakened after Bob had come in and given me a big hug. Jenn ran to greet Bob and immediately knew something was wrong. I could not tell her the news and Bob explained the diagnosis. Having no warning of bad news, she was in shock, and we hugged each other and cried. Bob called Chris to find out the details that I had forgotten.

Searching for something to do to help, Bob put the wheels in motion to get good medical advice from the States. During his trip there just ten days earlier, he had met Dr. Ken Block, director of the Pentagon health clinic. Bob immediately called Ken, explained the situation, and asked with whom we could consult at the Walter Reed Army Medical Center. Within an hour, Dr. Dave Jaques, chief surgeon at Walter Reed, called us at home. I strained to hear Dr. Jaques' soft and reassuring voice, and his information and assistance reassured me of his knowledge and concern.

The exact sequence of events blurs, but I know that one of the doctors in the States called Chris at home for his assessment of the lab report. During the course of the evening, I began to understand the options open to me. The doctors understood the terminology that I didn't, and they explained what it all meant and what various forms of treatment might be recommended. Dr. Jaques provided his home phone number and asked me to keep him informed as we learned more so we could consult on treatment options. He welcomed me to come to Walter Reed if I wanted treatment in the U.S.

That night, I cried and cried and cried. I felt terribly scared—of the unknown, the expected pain, the extent to which it might have spread, the amount of time I might be out of commission, the possibility it might be incurable. I worried about being in a Belgian hospital without fluency in the language, missing important events for the family over the holidays, and missing both family and business events in the coming months. Jenn came to tell me good night, and she cried. Bob held us both. What else could one do?

I thought only, "I don't want to die!" I could not stand the thought of not seeing the girls marry, have children, be successful and happy in life.

At that point, I was incapable of thinking of life. I had to work through the pain of facing death first. Bob held me most of the night, and neither of us slept well.

We decided not to tell anyone else until after the holidays, wanting to celebrate Chirstmas and Ashley's sixteenth birthday on December 29 without the burden of unhappines. Despite the decision being for the best, the days passed slowly and ominously. Holding that devastating news filled us with loneliness and dread.

On our twenty-seventh wedding anniversary, the day after the diagnosis, I choked on the words, "Happy anniversary." For years, I had dreamt of celebrating our fiftieth anniversary together. Neither set of our parents had that joy. I had spent all our married life silently recognizing when we passed significant landmarks that my parents had not shared. When all our children passed the age I was when Daddy died, I rejoiced. When Bob and I passed the ages and the last anniversary that my parents shared, I breathed a sigh of relief. I worried about Bob because his family also had a history of heart disease. And now, I was the one with a serious illness.

I longed to say to Bob, "I want to be married to you for fifty years." But, I could not voice the words because I was too scared that I wouldn't make it.

Somehow we made it through that weekend. We did normal things. We shopped, and I could hardly stand to talk to people when we met someone we knew.

"Do I look different?" I asked Bob. I certainly felt different.

"No, you look fine," he reassured. "Only your eyes are red."

We attended a Christmas reception at the home of friends, and I felt very fragile. I asked Bob not to leave me alone. We finished our Christmas decorating by putting away whatever wasn't already in place. And we gladly accepted a last-minute invitation to share Christmas dinner with Navy friends. They thought they were saving us from being alone without Kennon and Howard coming to visit. They were really giving us a chance to feel normal.

On Monday, December 23, Chris called with options for going to Jules Bordet Cancer Institute. It proved difficult to get anyone's attention over the holidays. The earliest we could be seen was Monday, December 30, a whole week away. Medically, waiting for a week posed no threat as most breast cancer is slow-growing. But, psychologically, it seemed like forever. I wondered how we could make it for that long with the knowledge that cancer had invaded my body and we were not doing anything about it. Chris offered to accompany us to meet the surgeon and render his professional opinion.

That night, I called my friend, Rhonda, who had been a sorority sister at the College of William and Mary thirty years earlier. Rhonda had breast cancer in 1993, having a mastectomy and immediate reconstruction. I found her at home in Louisville. Upset to hear my news, she talked to me at length about options and her own experience.

"Breast cancer is not a death sentence!" she reiterated until I could hear her message.

She explained her surgery, her reconstruction, the chemotherapy and its side effects. She was gentle, hopeful, and thorough, and I felt bad that I hadn't been there for her when she was having her treatment. The best resource, she thought, was *Dr. Susan Love's Breast Book*. She promised to send it express mail the next day. Despite the busy requirements of Christmas season, that's exactly what she did. What a friend.

With the diagnosis of breast cancer, I prayed as hard as I had ever prayed in my life. Although Episcopalian by faith, I felt too tired and fragile to attend the Anglican midnight service. The Catholic chaplain graciously welcomed us to the early evening service, and we tearfully prayed on Christmas Eve among our unknowing Catholic friends.

When we called Sarah on Christmas morning, she demanded, "What do you mean by your vague message about more tests?!"

I came as close to lying at that point as I ever had. "I'm doing okay, sweetheart, but I have some more tests as part of my physical." Then I changed the subject.

Much to our surprise, Christmas Day was enjoyable. Ashley, as always, had enough energy for the whole family. Since she did not know about the cancer secret, she kept us all hopping and laughing. We opened Christmas presents at home, shared a wonderful dinner with Nancy and Bill, and talked to all the family in the States.

The next few days dragged by. Rhonda's information suggested questions I needed to ask. Bob and I searched on-line for cancer resources. The issue of reconstruction troubled me. Rhonda had a TRAM-flap procedure where tissue from the stomach is tunneled up to construct a new breast. Subsequent surgery creates a nipple, and a tattoo images an areola. It sounded awful. Yet, with all the controversy about implants, I knew I didn't want any foreign substance in my body.

On December 29, Ashley's sixteenth birthday, we planned a surprise party at a local Belgian restaurant. It turned out to be a great success and she seemed completely surprised. I could tell by our near-failure, however, that Bob was distracted. Scheduled to pick up the guests and meet us at the restaurant, he made the excuse that he had to go to his office for weekend work. Jenn, Ashley, and I arrived late at the restaurant, expecting the guests to shout their surprise to Ashley. When we arrived, however, we saw empty tables. An hour later, a chagrined Bob showed up with teenage girls in tow. Mistaking the pick-up time by an hour, he admitted his thoughts were as scattered as mine. We pulled it off anyway, and a good time was had by all.

Telling Ashley that we had a meeting in Brussels on Monday, we picked up Chris Georgantopoulos on his day off, and the three of us drove to Brussels. *Dr. Susan Love's Breast Book* had arrived just that day from Rhonda, and I leafed through it while we drove to Brussels. It saved me from having to make conversation. Rhonda's note, written on December 23, was touching:

> *Dear Barbara,*
>
> *This will be a Christmas that you will never forget. But I feel confident that you will have many, many more years—many, many more Christmases—in which you will be able to reflect on the meaning of what happened this Christmas.*
>
> *I think my worst moments occurred when I was at the surgeon's office and he told me the results of the biopsy. But I quickly decided that I was not ready to die. And I didn't believe that it was my time. You probably have already gone through the hardest part. The pain from surgery and effects of any other treatment will be manageable because you know you are a survivor.*
>
> *I could tell you so many stories about women with breast cancer. These are stories that would have had no meaning for me four years ago. But things change. Life presents us with new challenges.*
>
> *My friends were so wonderful to me when I went through this. I needed them because I didn't have a husband and children. You are lucky to have them, and you should not hesitate to let them be the strong ones and take care of you for a few months. It's only temporary. You'll be back in control again in a short time. Then you'll find that people depend on you even more. They will assume you*

are the strong one who can handle anything if you got through this.

The bookstore had one copy of this new edition of Susan Love's book. Before mailing, I've been reading it for the latest development and discoveries. As I read it, I once again feel a sense of calm. She is very honest and so knowledgeable and therefore very comforting. She doesn't tell you what to do. But she explains all the options.

After you have seen the specialist, I hope that you don't feel compelled to make a quick decision. Hopefully you will feel that you have all the time you need to make your decision.

If there is any way I can help you, please call me. Sometimes it helps just to talk. You will be in my prayers.

Love,
Rhonda

The day was bitterly cold and we got hopelessly lost in Brussels as we tried to find the Jules Bordet Cancer Institute. We finally found it and parked some distance away. As we walked into the clinic, I shivered, held tightly to Bob and Chris, and tried not to fall on the uncharacteristic Belgian snow and ice. On entering the building, we were still confused about how to proceed and where to go for the appointment. Thank God for Chris. His fluent French eased the process in the new and strange clinic. We waited only a few minutes until we were called by a short lady in scrubs, Dr. Dina Hertens.

Dr. Hertens spoke excellent English. Direct and matter-of-fact, yet gentle, she read the lab reports and looked at the mammograms. The biopsied area clearly showed a tumor, she confirmed. The second suspicious area was less clear. She believed it might be a trick of the mammography, where two different views overlapped and created a shadow. During an actual exam, she palpated the tumor. I wondered why the Air Force physician who examined me just six weeks earlier hadn't felt something. She found no swelling in the lymph nodes, which she considered a good sign.

Chris, Bob, and I all liked her immediately. Although we had only booked a consultation, we nonverbally agreed that we needed to proceed with Dr. Hertens. I wanted the surgery as soon as possible, but again, the holidays presented a timing problem with New Year's Eve the next day. Dr. Hertens could get me a bed beginning Thursday, January 2, but surgery was less clear. She wanted the plastic surgeon available in the event of reconstruction, and the plastic surgeon was on vacation. Before I decided about reconstruction, I wanted to talk to the plastic surgeon. So, we agreed that I would check in to the hospital on January 2 for tests and consultation with the plastic surgeon. Surgery would be either Friday or Monday. Without knowing that, I must come prepared to stay.

Dr. Hertens' surgical nurse instructed me about hospitalization in Belgium and gave me material to read about Jules Bordet. As I waited for scheduling and information, I tried to control my tears. Bob stood behind me with his hand on my shoulder. Chris told me how well I was doing. Their support was vital, but I still felt very alone. It was a long ride back home from Brussels.

On our return home, we told Ashley right away. Sitting in the family room, I said, "Ashley, we need to tell you why we went to Brussels today."

She immediately sensed that things were not good. Her eyes darted back and forth from Bob to me.

"What's wrong?" she asked.

"Honey, I've been diagnosed with breast cancer and I'll go into the hospital on Thursday for surgery."

Her eyes filled with tears, "But you'll be okay, Mommy. I know you'll be okay!"

I had planned to chaperone her Model United Nations trip to The Hague in late January, and she said, "You'll be just fine and you'll still be able to go with us."

"I don't think so, Ash," I responded, but she would hear none of it. In fact, she was acting out her denial of such bad news.

On January 1, we shared the news with my sister, Kennon, and my mother. I called Kennon in Chicago first. After cheery greetings of Happy New Year, and questions about how Howard was recovering from his surgery, I told Kennon I had breast cancer. She immediately started to cry. Her world seemed to be crumbling with her husband and her sister both diagnosed with cancer.

"You should have a mammogram and an ultrasound as soon as possible," I told her. "Sisters of women with breast cancer are at risk."

We cried together and I shared my fears with her. As a clinical psychologist, she knows how to comfort, when to listen, and is good at interpreting what she hears.

Next, I called my mother. I had forgotten that she and my stepfather had company for New Year's in their Naples, Florida, winter home. She eagerly told me about their celebration and their friends. I told her I had bad news, which she listened to calmly and dry-eyed. She asked about our next steps and whether I needed her to come to Belgium. She offered to be on the next plane if I needed her, as I knew she would. We decided to wait a few days and see how the surgery went. She was encouraging and cited friends who had had breast cancer and were doing fine today. I learned later that it was only after we hung up that she felt the impact of the shock and broke down and cried.

Exhausted emotionally from those two calls, I decided not to call anyone else. Unsure whether I would stay in the hospital on January 2, we would wait before telling the rest of the family and friends. However, my business colleagues needed to know right away. Although living in Belgium, I served as chief executive officer of VIMA International, a leadership consulting firm headquartered in Virginia. Since 1988, VIMA had assisted clients in the United States and internationally. One week a month found me at company headquarters. From Belgium, I telecommuted and maintained daily contact with VIMA staff and clients. VIMA offices reopened on January 2 after a ten-day Christmas break.

I wrote a message to be presented at their staff meeting.

Happy New Year.

I hope you've all had a wonderful and restful break between Christmas and the New Year. It certainly is a time for re-energizing and spending time with family and friends. While you are now gearing up to get underway for the new year, I'm a bit under the weather. I didn't tell you or my family until today because I didn't want to dampen anyone's holidays. On December 10, I had a questionable mammogram, followed by two biopsies. On December 20, I learned that I have breast cancer. On January 2, I'll enter the Jules Bordet Cancer Institute in Brussels for treatment. The mammograms and ultrasounds are not conclusive, but we're keeping a positive outlook on the questions that the surgeon and pathologist still have.

The Belgian system is quite different from the U.S. system. On January 2, I'll have a myriad of tests: chest x-ray, bone scan, liver ultrasound, uterine ultrasound, EKG, blood work, urinalysis, and others I can't even remember. If all those tests come out okay, I'll have surgery on Friday, January 3 or Monday, January 6. The extent of the surgery will be determined while I'm asleep, so I have no more decisions to make. There is one certain invasive malignancy and one questionable area. Post-operative treatment will be determined after the surgery—either radiation, chemotherapy, or both. I will be in the hospital from seven to ten days.

Bob will be checking e-mail and bringing it to me in the hospital, so please keep me in the loop. It will help me to focus on something other than myself. I've talked twice to the head surgeon at Walter Reed who says I'll probably get bored in the hospital for seven to ten days. I hope so.

I will surely need your prayers and all the positive karma you can send my way. This is all a bit frightening. Not only is there cancer invading my body, but I'm having treatment in a second language. Although the surgeon speaks excellent English, the nursing staff and other medical providers speak French or Flemish. This will be a real test of my language ability.

I know you will all keep VIMA running smoothly, and that is a relief to me. I count on your prayers and support. Talk to you soon.

> *Love,*
> *Barbara*

A Cultural Surgical Experience

On January 2, Bob and I left our home in Mons at 5:30 a.m. in the frigid cold, taking a train to Brussels to the Jules Bordet Cancer Institute. Driving in downtown Brussels was something we didn't know quite how to do, and we had been so lost trying to find Bordet with Dr. Chris Georgantopoulos the week before that we decided to take the train and not worry about parking. When we arrived at the Brussels Midi train station, we walked through a long tunnel to reach the city metro. The temperatures dipped to record-breaking numbers for Belgium, in the teens Fahrenheit and well below zero centigrade, and the wind whipped through the tunnel. We towed a suitcase with us, and I can not remember ever being so cold—and full of dread. I shook all over and had no adrenaline to keep me warm.

After two stops on the metro, we walked two blocks to Bordet. I felt like a block of ice. I reported to the Nuclear Medicine Clinic at 7 a.m. When we found the correct floor and ward, it was empty and the offices were dark. Bob and I stood outside the door for twenty minutes, shivering. We learned later that the heat in the entire hospital had been off the day before and the building hadn't quite warmed up yet. The clinic entrance was off a long circular ramp that flowed up the side of the building, so the wind whipped through it like a wind tunnel. Finally, someone arrived and checked me in. I drank a sweet liquid and was injected with radioactive isotopes for the actual bone scan to be done two hours later.

I reported next to Admissions to be registered into the inpatient surgical ward. Nothing is easy when trying to communicate in a second language. Bob and I both speak some French, but under this stress, it all left me. Thank God, Bob took over for me. As instructed, I brought my Belgian identity card, my passport, and the insurance papers from the U.S. Army health clinic. The woman in Admissions was not particularly friendly nor helpful. Unfortunately, this first encounter with her would not be our last. I wondered why such people were hired for positions where they must deal with sick people. The last thing a sick person needs is to deal with an unhelpful receptionist.

We were introduced to the strange Belgian custom that a woman is always registered by her maiden name for anything official. Therefore, I was admitted as Barbara Pate. I explained as best I could to the admissions clerk that my name was Glacel, all my medical records, mammograms, biopsies, and so forth were under Glacel, my insurance was under Glacel, that anyone calling the hospital to find me would ask for Glacel, but it simply did not matter. My Belgian identity papers said my *nomme de jeune fille* was Pate and that was that. What made it all the more ridiculous was that the Belgians could not even pronounce Pate.

The admissions clerk did not like the insurance papers we brought and requested payment. At that point, Bob's usually calm, take-charge demeanor vanished. He insisted on talking to someone who spoke English. The English-speaking supervisor accepted the insurance papers, apologized for the problem, and sent us on to the fifth floor to check in to the ward. It all seemed a bit *laissez faire* to me. I wondered if I had been physically incapacitated how they would have helped me with all these logistics.

On the fifth floor, a nurse expected me and showed us into a double room. The other woman in the room was in very bad shape. I wondered if she had stomach cancer. She had all kinds of awful tubes coming in and out of her with terrible stuff draining, and she made awful noises. She also had the television on full blast all the time. With the television mounted on my side of the room, I had no choice but to be subjected to Belgian soap operas. I wondered: Would I be able stand to spend a week in this room?

The day's schedule included a myriad of tests with a confusing process and timetable. No one told me the schedule or where I was to go. I only knew to report back to Nuclear Medicine two hours after the injections. So, Bob and I sat in my room until the time came, and then we took off for Nuclear Medicine. As we left the surgical ward, a nurse ran after us asking where we were going as we were supposed to be taken to Nuclear Medicine.

"We can find it ourselves," we said, promising to return to be available for the other tests when called.

The long day included a lot of waiting for whatever unknown would be next. At one point, lunch arrived and we were introduced to Belgian hospital food. In an otherwise very somber and depressing day, lunch provided some comic relief. Not feeling hungry, I offered Bob the cardboard-looking hospital meal. It was a paradox to me that any institution in Belgium, known for the best French cooking imaginable and with fantastic restaurants from family-run to luxury-style, could serve such unimaginative and dull food.

During the afternoon, I went to several different clinics with a young man whose only function seemed to be to guide patients from one clinic to another. On later occasions, I would see him wheeling people in wheelchairs or pushing stretchers. However, since I could walk, I followed him in what seemed like a silent game of "Follow the Leader." When we arrived at the various clinics, I never knew quite what to do. He would motion me to sit down and I would wait for someone to call me. Eventually, a person would come into the hall and say, "Madame Pat." How was I to know that was me? I could understand Madame Glacel, and maybe even Madame Pate if I thought about it twice. But, on some occasions, I had no clue that Madame Pat was I.

In the radiology and ultrasound clinic, I experienced another taste of Belgian immodesty while having a vaginal ultrasound. Breast cancer is sometimes associated with other female cancers, and this test would both examine and set a benchmark for future exams.

"Go into the dressing room, undress from the waist down, and come out into the examining room," I was told.

No drape, just walk into the examining room nude from the waist down. This seemed even more bizarre to me than the same procedure for the breast exams. But, I did as instructed. Worse than a pelvic exam, the ultrasound involved having an instrument inserted into the vagina and then rotated around internally while the technician read the screen and took photos. Afterward, the same immodest procedure in reverse: Walk back to the dressing room bare from the waist down.

I never knew what to do after each test. Sometimes the young man waited for me to go to another clinic. If he weren't there, I would find my way back through a maze of corridors to the Surgical Ward and wait for the next summons. At some point, a team of medical students came to examine me, take blood, and talk about my case. A plastic surgery resident came to visit with his box of props and photos to talk about postsurgical options, especially reconstruction.

At this point, we did not know whether I would have a lumpectomy or a mastectomy. That decision would be made during surgery. So, we had to go into surgery having already decided about reconstruction in the event a mastectomy was performed. Rhonda had explained to me the reconstruction she had undergone, the TRAM flap procedure. The Belgians would not perform a flap procedure until one year after initial surgery, however, as they felt it masked any possible recurrences of the initial cancer. The only option they offered was an implant.

Belgians found the Americans overly dramatic about the problems with silicone implants. The Belgians still used silicone implants as well as the dual-lupin implants, which had a silicone core surrounded by saline. I definitely did not want an implant. Cancer was serious enough without the risk of putting any foreign substance in my body, regardless of the argument about silicone's safety. During the preceding weeks, I had consulted with a plastic surgeon at Walter Reed, whom I thought a bit cavalier about the decision and the "ease" of the options. He thought it was ridiculous that the Belgians would not do a TRAM flap right away. Bob and I read statements on-line from women who had reconstruction and who had not. We talked about whether it would bother Bob for me to be lopsided. He emphatically explained that whatever I wanted, he wanted too. He wasn't into worshipping me just for my body.

Although I did not want reconstruction, Dr. Hertens encouraged it. For a woman as young as I, she explained, a mastectomy could affect me psychologically and limit what clothes I could wear. She explained that after a mastectomy, the chest is almost concave and, even with a prosthesis, there is a gap that is not filled. Nonetheless, I held my ground on no reconstruction.

Bob and I understood that surgery might be either Friday or Monday, depending on the availability of the plastic surgeon. Since I decided not to have reconstruction, it actually would not have mattered.

"You can change your mind right up until the end," Dr. Hertens encouraged, "and the plastic surgeon will be standing by." She hoped I would change my mind.

Finally, she came to our room late in the day, saying the plastic surgeon would not be available on Friday. "You can go home," she told us. "We'll see you back here on Sunday night for early morning surgery on Monday. I hope you can enjoy your weekend."

I repacked my personal belongings, got my weekend "leave" pass, and Bob and I retraced our steps in the bitter cold, towing the suitcase behind us. In the Brussels Midi station, the icy conditions absolutely chilled us as we waited nearly an hour. Exhausted, we rode the train home and were welcomed by Jenn while Ashley would be spending the night with a friend.

Friday brought its own crisis. Jenn awakened in the early hours of the morning with intestinal flu. I reacted as a mother, holding her head as she threw up in the bathroom. When I reached Chris Georgantopoulos at his office, he worriedly directed me, "Don't stay in the same room with Jenn, and do not touch any of her things. If you get sick, the surgery will have to be postponed!"

Without Bob or Ashley at home to help, I bundled up Jenn and took her to the clinic to see Chris. Not only did he give her medicine and warn about dehydration, he supplied a box of surgical masks so that Jenn's flu germs would not affect the rest of the family. We spent the evening watching television while wearing surgical masks that made us look a bit like the alien television character "Alf."

My brother-in-law, Howard, had had his surgery for colon cancer postponed at the last minute just the month before. The delay had upset him. My reaction differed. This free weekend left me feeling calm and happy. Despite Chris's worries, I was glad to take care of Jenn. She had been great at taking care of me in this terrible time. Her flu proved to last only twenty-four hours and no one else in the family became ill. On Saturday, we shopped and planned meals, since Jenn would be in charge of cooking. We spent some good family time together.

On Sunday afternoon, I did something special for each member of the family and this connected me to each of them. I ironed or sewed something for Bob, Jenn, Ashley, and even Sarah, though she was in Russia. These chores had been piled up for months while I lived a somewhat schizophrenic existence as a businesswoman in the United States and an Army wife in Belgium. Now it felt good to leave each family member with something done especially for them.

By coincidence, my Norwegian exchange sister, Bodil, called to say Happy New Year. I had lived with her family in Oslo, Norway, in 1966, and we have been very close ever since. I had tried to write them a note over the weekend, and I could not find the words to tell them what was happening. I was so grateful that Bodil called, and I could tell her over the phone and ask her to deliver the message to her parents. Bodil's husband had gone through surgery for a brain tumor some years before, so she could imagine what the family was feeling at the moment.

Anticipating the possibility that the surgery would be postponed, we had not informed anyone else in Belgium or the States about the diagnosis. This "found" weekend of free time was much happier since we did not have to talk to anyone about the cancer. Instead, I wrote letters to be mailed on Monday and composed an e-mail message to be sent just minutes before Bob and I walked out the door, returning to the hospital on Sunday night. I could not have stood to be there to receive phone calls from folks once they read the e-mail.

January 5, 1997

Dear family and friends,

Bob and I have agonized over how to give bad news to family, godparents, and close friends. In our introversion, we have found it easier to keep the bad news to ourselves. But, now I think we would find your prayers and support helpful. On December 20, I was diagnosed with breast cancer. I'll be having surgery on Monday, January 6 at the Jules Bordet Cancer Institute in Brussels. We don't know much more than that until the surgery is over. I opted for staying here because it's important to me to be close to the family. We'll let you know when we know more about the prognosis and future treatment. In the meantime, we welcome your prayers.

Love,
Barbara

Bob and I drove to Brussels to arrive by 7 p.m. When we arrived at the Surgical Ward, we discovered I was assigned to a different room. Thank goodness. I had no roommate, much to my delight. Bob stayed to get me settled, and then he returned to Mons, promising to be waiting when I returned from surgery the next morning. I spent the evening doing some committee work for the William and Mary Alumni Board. Jenn would be able to take my work back with her. Again, I felt good about not leaving any loose ends.

The evening before surgery was full of not-so-pleasant procedures that we accomplished. Although I rarely take anything to help me sleep, I requested something that night. The anesthesiologist had to order it, and he would come talk to me before surgery. By 10 p.m., no one had come, so I called the nurse. She explained that the anesthesiologist had emergency surgery, and I should go ahead and turn off my light if I wished. At least, I think that is what she said. The Flemish-speaking nurses spoke a bit of English, but the French-speaking nurses spoke little. I realized that this hospital experience would definitely improve my French. The last thing I looked up in the dictionary before turning off the light was how to say "I need the bedpan, please."

I prayed a lot as I lay alone in the room wondering when the anesthesiologist would come. The prayer must have calmed me, since I fell asleep. The next thing I knew, the anesthesiologist woke me at 2 a.m. Barely coherent, I talked with him about anesthesia for the surgery, and he gave me something to help me go back to sleep.

The nurses awakened me at 6 a.m. and asked me to bathe with a special disinfectant soap. Belgian hospitals don't provide all the amenities that American hospitals do, so I had brought my own towels, wash cloth, even drinking water. I learned later that I should have brought my own thermometer. Since I had not known to do that, they provided me one, and charged it on my bill. I bathed in the disinfectant while gazing out the large windows, wondering if anyone in the surrounding office buildings could see me. At that point, though, the passing thought hardly bothered me. The Belgian lack of modesty had become almost normal.

Surprised that the bathroom was full of towels, I used one of theirs rather than my own. I donned the surgical gown and returned to my room to await the next step. Given a pill to relax me, I waited to be taken to the surgical clinic. It felt strange to be wheeled on the stretcher down the corridor, into the elevator, past the long circular corridor where Bob and I had waited in the cold just four mornings ago, and into the surgical clinic. From that prone position, I found it hard to know who was who and to figure out the layout of the rooms and operating theaters. Since all the conversation flowed in French or Flemish, everything seemed even more surreal. I was "parked" by a wall for a while and wondered if anyone knew or cared if I were there.

Finally, Dr. Hertens came and introduced me to a very tall, blonde woman, the head of plastic surgery. Dr Hertens still hoped I would say yes to reconstruction. I had not changed my mind, and the plastic surgeon kindly said that was absolutely fine and completely up to me. I remember then being wheeled into the operating room, transferred to the operating table surrounded by several people in scrubs, and given an IV.

A bright light shining in my eyes slowly awakened me. Gradually, I became aware of voices around me. Something seemed to say to me that my breast had been saved. I still do not know whether Dr. Hertens told me that, whether I dreamt it, or how I knew. As I became more aware of the recovery room, I saw the sun shining in a window to my right side. Knowing that I would not be released from the recovery room until I could urinate, I asked the recovery room nurse for the *bessin de lit.*

All of this took a while, and moving my right side caused pain. I thought I spoke French, but the nurse talked to me in English. At one point the man next to me asked what we said, and the nurse laughingly responded, "It's just between us girls."

Finally, the recovery room released me and an attendant wheeled me back to my room. As we rolled down the long corridor, I raised my head a little and could see Bob waiting at the end of the hallway in the waiting room. By the time we turned into my room, he had arrived and reached for my hand. I noticed that I now had a roommate, but that was the least of my concerns at the moment. The transfer from the stretcher into the bed caused more pain, not in the breast area but under my arm where lymph nodes were removed. Apparently there is no way to remove the lymph nodes without causing major trauma to muscles and nerves. In fact, one is barely able to move the arm for several days and physical therapy is usually required to regain mobility.

I had a drain under the arm and still received IV fluids. The orders were not to get out of bed until the next day, and then only with assistance. This was so different from the same surgery in American hospitals, where "drive-by" mastectomies are performed. A typical hospital stay for a lumpectomy in the United States is one night; for a mastectomy, two nights. Patients go home with drains and have to measure their own fluid discharge and return to the doctor's offices for postsurgical procedures. I felt glad to have someone else taking care of my needs during these days.

Bob stayed with me as I dozed, moving in and out of consciousness all day. He had brought with him several e-mail messages that had come in response to the message we sent out the night before. Our friends and family expressed the same shock we had felt on learning the diagnosis. My eyes clouded as I read their positive messages of love and support.

As per our plan, Bob told three important people that morning what was happening. First, he told his assistant Liz and asked her to let others in his office know. Then he called the high school and talked to both the guidance counselor and the principal. Ashley was in a bit of denial, expressing concern that people might talk about her mother's breast. She wanted to know that everything would be fine, that her life would not be disrupted, and that we would not be inconvenienced by this setback.

Before Bob left for home that night, Dr. Hertens arrived. She explained that she had removed the lump and achieved clean margins around the tumor. She had done a needle biopsy through the breast to the second suspicious site. Both sections were rushed to the lab and preliminary tests came back that the margins were clean and the second site was not malignant. Therefore, she had performed breast conservation and not a mastectomy. She felt so pleased, and, of course, so were we. We would have the report on the lymph nodes by the end of the week when I was released.

Bob took the train back to Mons, knowing that he had many more phone calls to make that night. To each person, Bob gave the same message: "There is good news and bad news. The good news is that they got it all; the bad news is that Barbara had surgery today for breast cancer."

Bob called Sarah in Russia. She probably knew something was wrong because Bob rarely placed our calls to her, and this call had not been scheduled. In fact, he reached her on Three Kings Day, the day the Russians celebrate Christmas. Her reactions were quick and varied. Furious that we had not told her, and in fact had come close to lying to her, she was terrified that I would die. She felt lonely, being so far from home. And, she wanted to come home immediately. Bob assured her that I did not want her to do that, and that if anything were immediately life-threatening, we would have her come home. He promised that we would inform her of everything now that we knew what we were dealing with, and that I would call her the minute I returned home from the hospital. I'm sure all this notification and emotion completely drained him.

Back in Bordet, I rested a bit more comfortably but found it very difficult to move at all. I knew the nurses were busy getting people ready for bed, but all the IV fluids meant I needed the *bessin de lit* fairly often. When I could not wait any longer, I pushed the call button. No one came, and I pushed

26

again. Then I noticed that it had become disconnected. I could not move enough to reach the overhead electrical strip to reconnect it.

All afternoon, the curtain had been drawn between my roommate and me, but I had seen her walk back and forth to the bathroom several times. Her husband had also come to visit. They were a sweet older couple, probably in their late sixties or early seventies. They were quiet and did not watch the television. I knew now that salvation lay in this dear, sweet lady. I summoned up my best French and asked her to help me. She came across the room, plugged in my call button, and I summoned the *bessin de lit*, never so happy to have a roommate.

I slept off and on during the night. I took pain pills and a sleeping pill, but also made frequent calls for the *bessin de lit*. Sometimes, the nurse would leave me on it for a long time while she tended to others who needed her. Not very comfortable. My back ached terribly because I could not lie in any other position than on my back. The night seemed endless.

On Tuesday morning, I had trouble eating breakfast. I could not manage to do much with my right arm because of the pain from the lymph node dissection. I learned the morning hospital ritual. Two nurses arrived to change linens, take vital signs, and wash patients who could not do it themselves. I still had not been allowed out of bed, so a nurse gave me a sponge bath in bed. Ultimately, it felt better to be clean, but the bath represented another example of both Belgian immodesty and discomfort. Finally, by midmorning I walked to the bathroom by myself. What an event—dragging the IV pole, the drainage bottle, and trying not to hurt my right side. Still, it showed progress. And I realized that this experience would be more than a medical procedure; it was truly a cultural experience.

Beginning the Journey to Recovery

Bob arrived at midday on the day following surgery with more e-mail messages from friends and family. My spirits lifted to hear their concern and feel their thoughts and prayers flying across the miles. I felt relieved that the three weeks of holding that solitary secret were behind us. Although I am an introvert by nature, I know that I need to talk things out to get through them. It was therapeutic to be able to respond to those in my inner circle and tell them what the experience felt like. In fact, Bob managed to hook up my laptop to the phone system so that I could communicate on my own.

Bob also brought a book, *Joining the Club: The Reality of Breast Cancer* by Lillie Shockney. Lillie's brother and sister-in-law were stationed with us in Mons. The news of my diagnosis had traveled fast when Bob released it the day before. Lillie's sister-in-law, Mary, and I had planned to be the chaperones on the Model United Nations trip that Ashley was so certain I would not miss in late January. When Bob arrived at his office Tuesday morning, he found a note from Mary along with Lillie's book.

Mary wrote, "Bob's sister, Lil, has had breast cancer for nine years. Lil has written a book about her experiences and lectures frequently about her life. You'll love her book. It's uplifting, serious, gut-wrenching, and comical. I hope it helps you in some way."

By the time Bob left the hospital to take the train back home on Tuesday night, I thought I might eventually feel like recovering. Changing positions and getting out of bed caused discomfort, but the love and concern moving into my life created a positive force. I felt tired, but not sleepy, so I opened *Joining the Club*. Lillie Shockney's story sounded so familiar and reassuring that I simply continued to read until I had finished the whole book. She told stories that were comical even in the face of cancer. Within the first nine pages, Lillie had me both weeping and laughing over her friend Miss Bertha's prosthesis woes. Apparently Miss Bertha decided to take up golf to recover range of motion in her affected arm after surgery. Without the advantage of a mastectomy bra in those days, when Miss Bertha took a huge swing, the prosthesis fell right out onto the ground. And then there was Miss Bertha's friend who had a bilateral mastectomy. She decided on an inflatable bra that expanded and burst on an airplane flight.

If these courageous ladies could share their stories and laugh, there was hope for us all. What a blessing to be able to laugh! My spirits lifted immediately. I couldn't wait for Bob to arrive on Wednesday so he could read the first nine pages of the book. I immediately ordered copies for Mother and our daughters to read. I will always appreciate Mary's gift of the book and Lillie's gift of her experience which started me on the path of laughter to get through the coming months.

On Wednesday, mobility increased, but I still needed help with my sponge bath. I felt as though my body wouldn't straighten up. I stood doubled over in the bathroom while the nurse helped me wash. The physical therapist arrived to demonstrate exercises for my arm. Because the lymph node removal, called an axillary dissection, inevitably damages muscle and nerves, the affected arm loses mobility. I began wall climbing and hanging rotation exercises of my arm. The physical therapist massaged and exercised my arms and legs to avoid any thrombosis from being immobile in the hospital. By the time she left, I felt exhausted.

My roommate had surgery this day, leaving me happily alone in the room. Flowers arrived and the phone rang a few times, but the unusual frosty weather kept potential visitors at home. Bob and Jenn arrived after lunch, cheering me up. Somehow, putting on a happy face for one's child is a natural thing to do. We had told Ashley she could visit or wait until I came home from the hospital, and she decided to wait until I returned home, keeping her life as normal as possible.

All the girls were with me in spirit, though. That was important. Jenn had bought me a little red-hatted gnome at a Christmas market and asked that I keep him with me so he could watch over me. Sarah had knitted me slippers before she left for Russia, and they kept my feet warm. Ashley had put together a photo collage for me to have next to my bed, featuring happy pictures of Jenn, Ashley and Bob, Sarah and Ashley as little girls, and a family photo from Sarah's high school graduation that also included our Finnish exchange daughter, Keiju.

My little table of objects reminded me of my friend Max, who had died a year earlier of leukemia. When he had his most severe treatments, he arranged a table of symbols of his life that helped him focus on his will to live and on happier times. He had photos, statues, and a wonderful saying by Nathalia Crane:

You cannot choose your battlefield,
The gods do that for you,
But you can plant a standard
Where a standard never flew.

There was no question in my mind that Max had planted a firm standard. Although he ultimately lost his battle to leukemia, he lived another five years after his terminal diagnosis. He entered clinical trials and had painful experimental procedures in the search for a better treatment for himself and others. He continued to give of himself to his friends and his country. His battle was an inspiration to me, and I often thought that I would not want to disappoint him as I waged my own battle with cancer.

Dr. Jaques had told me that I would be bored with a long stay in the hospital. However, the time to myself helped and allowed me the opportunity to emotionally deal with the illness and treatment. By Thursday, the fifth day, I felt much better. I moved around more easily, I spent most of the day in a chair, and I did my own e-mail. The Belgian nurses were amazed. The aggressive American businesswoman who brings her computer to the hospital for cancer surgery portrayed a new phenomenon to them. For me, it provided a lifeline. The contact made me know that there was life after breast cancer and that, although I was many miles from home, I had the love and support of family and friends. Their expressions of concern inspired and motivated me to kick this disease.

Two special visitors on Thursday night made it a memorable day. Amazed, I saw Rose walking in the door. Her husband waited in the car, and I could hardly believe that they had driven from Mons in the dark, on treacherous icy roads. Rose gave me four gifts that night. First, she gave me *Chicken Soup for the Soul*. I had heard the title, but never read any of the uplifting stories written and compiled by Jack Canfield and Mark Victor Hansen. During the course of my treatment, I would ultimately receive several different *Chicken Soup* editions and I came to value the stories that "open the heart and rekindle the spirit." Second, Rose gave me a foot massage. I had never had a foot massage, and it felt a little awkward at first. I mean, who would want to touch somebody's sweaty feet? Her gift of touch and acceptance was a meaningful symbol as well as a relaxing massage. Third, Rose begged me not to get implants. She told me of specific problems with silicone implants that had burst. Despite the medical jury being out, a personal experience can be quite persuasive, and Rose wanted me to hear the story. Finally, Rose asked if she could pray with me. Happy with that gift, I also felt a bit awkward at first. Rose prayed beautifully for me, for my family, and for my caregivers. She spoke so naturally in her conversation with God, and she truly transferred a sense of calm.

Dr. Dina Hertens arrived as the other special visitor. Sometimes undeniable chemistry develops between two people. You both know that the other feels it, but you don't know why or how to describe it. Dr. Hertens and I had simply hit it off. From my first visit to her, I appreciated the honesty and directness she somehow combined with a caring and gentle manner. I often prefer women doctors, and she personified that blend of nurturing with professionalism that many women doctors provide naturally. She visited me at the end of her rounds, and we chatted for nearly thirty minutes. I learned a bit about her, her husband, also a physician, and their lives. We talked about their travel in the United States. I talked to her about *Dr. Susan Love's Breast Book* and Lillie Shockney's *Joining the Club* and promised to get her copies of both. In light of how my case was to unfold the next day, our sharing that night created a special trust and bond between us.

Dr. Hertens promised that if the drains came out on Friday, I could go home. But I was unprepared for the pain of removing them. It truly took my breath away, and I felt the sensation all the way to my fingertips as she removed the drain from the axillary incision.

When I could speak, I gasped, "Oh my gosh-have you ever had drains removed after surgery?"

"No," she admitted, "I have never had surgery."

"I have a suggestion. All medical school students should be required to have surgery and have drains removed before they do it to a patient. It hurts!"

Dr. Hertens asked me to stay all day in the hospital because the Tumor Board met in the afternoon. She would come immediately from that meeting to tell me what the committee of doctors said about my case. If all was well, I would be discharged Friday evening. Bob arrived in the afternoon, having left instructions for Jenn to fix a "welcome home" dinner. Chris Georgantopoulos arrived in late afternoon, hoping to see Dr. Hertens and hear the report firsthand. Finally, our friend Becky arrived for a visit, not knowing that I might be going home that day. We waited and waited, but no Dr. Hertens. Chris finally left at 6 p.m. to return to his family in Mons and asked us to call him about the report of the Tumor Board. We sat with Becky until almost 7 p.m., when the nurse told us we might as well check out since Dr. Hertens had been held up.

Bob and Becky ferried the flowers and my belongings out to the car and were helping me on with my coat when Dr. Hertens ran up the hall. She apologized and said quickly, "I need to talk to you."

While Becky waited, we went to the lounge with Dr. Hertens. Clearly distraught, she gave us the news. The pathology reports came back showing that the second site was, in fact, malignant. One lymph node had been positive. This news reversed the optimism we had felt all week.

The protocol for two sites of breast cancer is clear: mastectomy. Dr. Hertens, however, wanted us to understand other options. She explained that with lumpectomy, one undergoes radiation to the rest of the breast. The radiation is designed to kill exactly the size cancer cells that had been discovered at the second site. If we had not biopsied the second site, we wouldn't know that surgery was recommended. She knew I didn't want reconstruction, and she wanted so much to conserve the breast. She pleaded with me to either forego a mastectomy and have radiation or to have reconstruction with the mastectomy. She felt it to be so important for a woman as young as I to have a complete body. She admitted that she was probably overstepping the bounds of the doctor-patient relationship, but she wanted me to consider her advice.

Stunned by all this news, I found myself calmly saying that I would think about it over the weekend and call her the following week.

"I don't blame you for this bad news, Dr. Hertens," I told her. "And I appreciate your concern and all you have done for me this week."

With that, Bob and I silently walked down the hall, gathered up Becky, and left the hospital for our cold drive home.

The Good News and the Bad News

It was good to be home, but we all felt a bit discouraged. The next day, I sent a message entitled "Good news and bad news."

January 11, 1997

Dear friends,

The good news is that I am writing this from home. I was released from the hospital on Friday, earlier than expected. The doctor was pleased with the surgical healing. I got home about 8 p.m. Friday night and enjoyed the best meal I had tasted in a week—frozen cannelloni with bottled tomato sauce. The hospital food was typical institutional food with even less creativity. Breakfast was two pieces of dry wheat bread with jam or honey. Lunch was the hot meal of the day, always something with a thick, cholesterol-full, fattening sauce. Dinner was two pieces of dry wheat bread with mystery toppings. We made it into a game to guess what the mystery would be before we took the lid off—cold cuts, cheese, tuna, grated carrots, pickled onions or something like that.

I was lucky to have the sweetest little lady as a roommate. Her name was Susan. She was probably in her late sixties and she had had surgery for breast cancer six years ago, now in the hospital for a hysterectomy. Both of us spent lots of time reading instead of having the blaring French soap operas that our neighbors had (and we could hear without being in their room). I managed to get along pretty well in French, although one day I gave the right answer to the wrong question. I thought they asked if I wanted help with my

33

"toilette." Since I couldn't move my right arm well, I answered yes. I found out later they asked if I had been able to go to the "toilette" yet. Well, right answer anyway.

As I was being discharged about 6:30 Friday night, the doctor finally appeared. Apparently the breast cancer team had been meeting all afternoon and struggling with my case. The doctor raced down the hall to catch me before I left. The bad news is that there is more cancer they didn't take out with the lumpectomy. The original biopsy while I was in surgery didn't reveal it. But subsequent tests over the five days revealed the growth of more cancer cells. The doctor is as distraught as I am. I have every confidence in her, and I feel like we are "in this together." There are two options for further treatment, and we're back to the drawing boards for more decision-making. There was also some minor lymph node involvement, so a systemic treatment is indicated. One treatment is a pill called tamoxifen that I would take for five years. We won't know if I can take that for another week or so when more lab results come back. I return to the hospital next Thursday to get stitches removed, and we will decide on what will follow, to begin within the next week.

So, for the moment, we're spending a very cold and somewhat discouraging weekend at home. Bob has begun training for his second career by washing my hair, and he has rigged up a rope pull to help me get out of the water bed. I'm continuing the physical therapy exercises for my arm, and hope my mobility returns very soon. Jenn leaves tomorrow to go back to William and Mary, and we will miss her. She is such a huge help. Ashley has exams next week, so the stress is on for her. My mother arrives on Friday, and we're thankful she is coming to help us. We are having our New Year's reception on Saturday with about 200 people. Mother, Bob and the caterer will pull that off, and I intend to "receive" as if I were the queen.

Thanks for your continuing prayers and love.

Barbara

While I tried to put an optimistic spin into my message, we all felt pretty low. Jenn did not want to return to college and offered to stay back to take care of me.

"That's not an option," I told her. "You have a life too!"

Mother arranged to come to Belgium at the end of the week, as much to help with our traditional command New Year's reception as to take care of me. Being surrounded by lovely flowers and receiving uplifting e-mail messages helped me face the discouragement that surrounded us. But in truth, I felt very down.

As I entered this unknown cancer journey, my sister became my strongest support, even as she coped with her husband's cancer. Her willingness to listen, analyze, and accept my feelings offered a much-needed outlet. As our e-mail messages became more frequent, we reverted to our childhood nicknames for each other, KP and BP. This message was appropriately titled "Some days are shit."

January 13, 1997

Dear BP,

It's now 5:20 in the afternoon and I am just getting back to writing to you. Howard was at the doctor's for an hour and a half, then I took him to his friend's architecture office for the rest of the day. He didn't want to come home to just sit and think about the first chemo injection. I read your e-mail to Mother so I know that you have decided to have the mastectomy and frankly that makes me happy. The emphasis made by each doctor that Howard has seen is that there is no guarantee that chemotherapy takes care of all the cancer cells. That's why there is a statistic given to Howard that without chemotherapy he has a fifty-fifty chance of no more cancer and with chemotherapy he has a 75 percent chance. So even with chemotherapy there is a 25 percent chance that cancer cells will be able to hide from the drugs.

I would guess that radiation is the same—there are no guarantees. Therefore you would want to take out of the body any cancer that you know is there. I also do not believe that anything happens by chance. So I would say that it was not chance that the surgeon biopsied the other area, only to discover some days later cancer cells growing in the tissue. She may wish she had not done the biopsy but I am glad she did and the result requires more action than radiation.

As for reconstruction surgery, it is most important that you know yourself to answer this question. There would be no question for me. I would not have it and I would wear something on the out-

side. Probably knowing me I would wear an undershirt and forget about it. But that's me. I do not trust putting foreign objects in my body, I would not want my stomach tissue to have a new job, and I want as little surgery as I can have. Your surgeon, I will bet, would take the opposite position for herself and that is what she was really telling you by talking about the feelings of other women patients. So you must listen to these different opinions and then think what is true and right for you. I'll support whatever you decide to do. I just want the cancer out of you.

Over the next week I'm going to put together a package of things for you, a CARE package. Also I'm going to call and e-mail—as much as you can stand—just so you know I'm fighting this with you. Think of the cancer as Samuel and I'm on the way down the street to beat him up. Just thinking of it as Samuel is enough to do everything to get rid of it. Well, BP, it is 12:45 AM for you and hopefully you are sleeping peacefully and tomorrow will be a better day. But don't worry when you have bad days, give me a call and we'll cry together.

I love you,
Kennon

Her reference to Samuel really made me laugh. Samuel lived down the street from us when we were children. As the youngest of three children, I always had my older brother and sister to take up for me. One time when I whined that Samuel was picking on me, Kennon rode her bike down the street, prepared to beat him up. I don't remember the outcome of that encounter and, of course, we were all friends again within a short period of time, but the image of Kennon at age fifty riding her bike down the street to beat up my cancer was a great boost.

Another good laugh came from Becky in her message entitled "*Toilette.*"

You got along extremely well with the French. I am so proud of you. Your story of the toilette is logical. When I was eighteen having a tonsillectomy, I was the oldest tonsillectomy patient (the rest were all six to eight) and having a rough go of it. By the time I got out of surgery, the other kids were eating ice cream. I wasn't. I wanted none of that. They finally moved me out of pediatrics into an adult ward, but did so while the family was at supper. They came back, my bed was empty and remade. I like to think they got upset and asked what happened, but I think they knew because they found me with no difficulty.

Anyhow, the nurse came by and asked if I had had a BM. No, I said, I had my tonsils out. (And this is in ENGLISH). She left, I realized my mistake, but felt too bad to correct it. What a gas. Hospitals. So your French double-talk wasn't bad at all.

On Thursday, Bob drove me to Brussels to have the stitches removed from the lumpectomy and the axillary dissection. Unable to bathe all week, I had washed a little with sponge baths.

After removing the stitches, the nurse put antiseptic spray on the areas and I gasped, "It stings!"

Laughing, Dr. Hertens said, "Of course, you haven't washed all week."

It took me a minute to realize that Dr. Hertens thought I had said, "It stinks!" It probably did, but somehow explaining all that wasn't worth the energy of translation.

I still had such limited mobility in my arm that I asked the nurse to fasten my bra for me. Despite doing the exercises at home, I knew that the next surgery would set me back on regaining mobility. I scheduled the next surgery for January 21 and went through the instructions again for admittance.

The cultural differences of receiving cancer treatment in Belgium became more obvious as we moved into this phase. We learned that a Belgian doctor could lose the license to practice by telling a patient that the patient's illness could be terminal. The prevailing medical philosophy stated that patients did not need to know the details of the illness. The doctors were the decision-makers, and patients did not involve themselves with decisions on treatment. Luckily, Dr. Hertens did not ascribe to this philosophy. She explained to me the options, gave her opinion, but accepted when I wanted to be more conservative, as in requesting a mastectomy and declining reconstruction.

However, as we began talking about next steps, things became more difficult. The Tumor Board decided on follow-on treatment, and patients were expected to follow their recommended protocol. Because I had decided on the mastectomy, no breast tissue remained for radiation therapy.

With even one positive lymph node, I expected to receive chemotherapy. However, for post-menopausal women, the Belgian protocol did not call for chemotherapy. If my tumor proved to be estrogen-receptor positive, I would receive only tamoxifen, a chemo-by-pill that is taken for five years. As I understood it, the tamoxifen typically, but not always, acted as an estrogen receptor antagonist in the breast. The tamoxifen binds available estrogen receptors on breast cells, and thus prevents estrogen from binding. This, in turn, prevents estrogen from stimulating the development of more breast cancer cells.

There were, of course, advantages and disadvantages to tamoxifen. It would provide similar benefits to estrogen, reducing the rate of heart attack and stabilizing bone loss that could lead to osteoporosis. The side effects, however, could include hot flashes, weight gain, an increased susceptibility to uterine cancer, depression, eye problems, phlebitis, and pulmonary problems.

On the surface, the tamoxifen sounded like a good trade-off to me—much easier follow-on treatment and I would not lose my hair. But as I did more reading, I became uneasy with that protocol absent chemotherapy. I felt confused and wondered how I might be treated in the United States for this medical condition. Dr. Jacques at Walter Reed had cautioned from the beginning that I was too young to be treated medically as post-menopausal. This raised many questions for me.

In just two weeks, the word had spread far and wide about my cancer. Although I heard from friends, I felt a void in personal contact and touch. I realized that our many wonderful NATO friends simply did not know what was culturally acceptable in the face of serious personal problems. They did not know whether they should talk about cancer or not. Those who knew me well enough to want to talk sometimes did not speak enough English to express their own support and fear. I realized then that my support group would be mostly those folks who were afar and communicated by e-mail and mail.

January 17, 1996

Dear family and friends,

I appreciate all your good wishes and prayers. Forgive me for not answering each message, but know that your messages to me are received gratefully. I had the stitches out yesterday and feel better today. I have the weekend to gear up for round two. On Monday, I'll be re-admitted to Jules Bordet Cancer Institute for more surgery. Again, I'll be in the hospital for about six days. We still don't know what the follow-on treatment will be.

Mother arrived this morning, is already unpacked and taking a nap. I am so glad she is here. It seems that no matter how old one is, having a mom around when you're sick is super. Next week will be a juggling act, but that's nothing new for this family. Ashley will be in The Hague for five days for the Model United Nations conference. Bob has to be in England for three days. Mother will stay in Brussels with friends so she can get to the hospital more easily. And, of course, Jenn is back in Williamsburg and Sarah still in Russia. Both of them feel very far away at a time when the comfort of family is important.

For the weekend, we're just concentrating on our New Year's reception that will be tomorrow. The caterer has just been here to deliver glassware, ice, plates, coat rack, etc. He assures me that I have nothing to worry about. So, I'll enjoy the champagne and good company.

Thanks for your prayers.

Love,
Barbara

The reception boosted my spirits and made me glad we held it. Bob had asked if we should cancel it, but the invitations had gone out long before I knew about my cancer diagnosis. I thought it would make me feel worse to cancel it than to go ahead and have it, even if I could not be a very active hostess. As it turned out, though, I stood for most of the evening and greeted each guest at the door. Some guests knew that I had just had surgery and others didn't. We didn't dwell on it, but I didn't mind talking about it either. The NATO Commanding General arrived, and in his eagerness to express his concern for me, he gave me a huge squeeze. His thoughtfulness was great, but my sore and fragile body suffered for it.

A friend had spent the whole afternoon arranging flowers for the tables, and I thought that maybe my being sick had some advantages. Our house would never have looked so elegant without the help of talented and loving friends. One disappointment, though, came when I confided to an

American friend that I had just gotten out of the hospital having had surgery for breast cancer. She gave a small sympathetic response, but I never heard from her afterwards. I was so disappointed that, despite my need for support from those close-at-hand, she did not respond to me. I surely never felt the same toward her again. I did not believe anyone owed me care and concern. Simply, I craved support, and physical touch, and longed for someone else's strength to help see me through this difficult time. I longed for others to reach out.

"Barbara, the Protestant congregations are praying for you and your recovery," the chaplain said as he left the reception.

Moved, I thanked him tearfully. "I know we're doing the right thing with the second surgery," I said. "I feel a true sense of calm and peace, and all the prayers must be the reason."

American friends were the last to leave. Nancy and Candace would prove to be generous and helpful friends in the weeks ahead. They shopped for me and took my mother wherever she needed to go during her stay. Nancy often made dinners for me during the coming months of treatment. I welcomed these American friends who understood that the usual support of an American military installation did not exist in the international community. I dispensed all the flowers to Nancy, Candace, and the catering crew. Since I was to reenter Jules Bordet in two days, there was no reason to waste the flowers on an empty house. I saw the tears in the eyes of the Belgian servers who had done many parties in our home, and I appreciated their silent concern. But I was ready to go on and get this cancer out of my body. I truly felt everyone's support, and I was going into this surgery with an amazing sense of calm. Surely, my life was more important than any body part, and I wanted to get on with it.

Vulnerability

As I started round two of surgery, I realized that it felt so much easier now that others knew my situation. I felt wrapped in a cocoon of love and prayers. I had prayers being offered by many people whom we had known during a mobile Army career. My hometown church and the churches of friends and family included me in their prayers. Our Jewish and Muslim friends offered prayers in their own traditions.

I gratefully accepted every prayer and positive thought in any form it was offered. As a high-control person who is used to being in charge, I found it difficult to let go and allow others to take over for me. One of the reasons I turned down several offers of family and friends to come to Belgium to care for me was that I knew I would want to be in charge, be the hostess, and take care of them.

Instead, I struggled with feeling so vulnerable. One person who had seldom reached out to me before seemed to gush all over me with good wishes, which I experienced as irritating and insincere. I wondered if I had now become more acceptable to this person because I had shown a flaw in my otherwise steady exterior.

Another friend seemed to capture this issue of vulnerability in her letter. Her explanation made sense to me.

> *I have only glimpsed your emotional side, and I believe this is because your personality is so strong that you do not allow others to see an unsure, or vulnerable Barbara. We all experience times when the earth seems not very solid under our feet. Our faith in God and courage at those times support us and allow us to do all that is*

important and necessary. In my heart, I know you have all the right attributes to be a successful victor. This disease will simply be one more challenge to overcome. You will, as a result, be an even stronger and more wonderful human.

When I felt down, I communicated less and that worried my e-mail support group. While I felt lonely being so far away from friends and family, they were also suffering in not being able to be with me. They needed information about me as much as I needed information about cancer and treatment options. As I entered the hospital for the second surgery, one friend answered my message saying:

Thanks for your message. I needed it worse than you need support from me. Doesn't mean that I'm withdrawing any support, just wanted you to know that I appreciate your messages and thoughts.

On Monday, January 20, Bob took me back to Jules Bordet Cancer Institute. He and Mother settled me in the room and then he took Mother to Randy and Becky's where she would stay for three days. Bob had business in England that had been scheduled for some time, and I persuaded him that it would be all right for him to go. Almost as soon as he left, I regretted telling him to go. Had I wanted him to stay, he would have canceled the trip, but my insistence freed him to go. I had not allowed myself to be weak and simply say, "I'm scared and I want you with me." I wrote to him before I went to sleep that night:

January 20, 1997 from the hospital

Hi Sweetheart,

It is 9 o'clock and I decided to set up the computer. I feel more like doing it tonight than I will after the surgery. My roommate's name is Bridgette. She has been here for five days and she said how lucky I am to have Dr. Hertens. Her level of English is about the same as my level of French, so we should do okay. I love you so much. Please be careful and come back to me soon. I really need you to get through the months ahead.

Love,

B

I completed the same presurgery routine to prepare the night before and the morning of surgery. As I had my antiseptic bath, I discovered much to my dismay that this time the bathroom had no towels and I had not brought one from home. What a challenge to dry my entire body with the two tiny wash cloths I found. As I entered the operating room, Dr. Hertens gave me one last chance to select reconstruction, and again I declined. By now, it had become a bit of a joke between us, and she realized I was a strong-willed American. She took that in good stride, and I again felt grateful for her skills and her empathy.

I woke up in the recovery room and immediately realized I was on the opposite side of the room from my first surgery. I think that made such an impression on me because the sun again blazed in the large windows and I lay right in the path of its rays. I felt very hot and uncomfortable. The nurses were loud and laughing, and it all annoyed me. I couldn't seem to get anyone's attention to ask for the *bessin de lit* or once I got it, to get them to take it away. I just wanted to get out of there. The pain seemed much more immediate than it had after the first operation, although I would discover that the recovery would be faster because the lymph node dissection had been done with the first surgery.

Finally, the orderly wheeled me back to my room and I found Mother anxiously waiting. Feeling grateful that she was there, I still missed Bob terribly. She spent the afternoon with me while I dozed, and Becky came to pick her up at 6:30.

Distraught that she could not be in Belgium during this time, Jenn felt very alone and far away. As soon as I felt able, I sent her my first e-mail message:

January 22, 1997

Hi Sweetie,

It is Wednesday afternoon and Nanna has pulled my e-mail at the hospital. I am feeling a little better today. Yesterday and last night were awful. I had a lot of pain and got nauseated. Today I'm feeling more like myself. I have on my green Victoria Secret pajamas. I'm so glad you talked to Sarah. Because both of you are far away, you can reassure each other. Daddy called last night from England and will call again tonight. I can't wait for him to get back. I really missed his being here for this operation, but Nanna has been wonderful.

I love you lots, Babe. I miss your chocolate chips.

Love,
Mommy

Dear Mommy,
I'm so glad to hear from you. It has been very sad to have no e-mails from you, but I got one from Dad that was very exciting. Lots of people send their love. I talked with Sarah last night. She had a hard day on Tuesday, but was so glad to hear everything was fine. She says to tell you she loves you and misses you lots. She was wearing all black so I made her promise to put on one bright thing at least. My New Year's resolution is to wear and buy bright clothes.
Today has been a good day. I think that just knowing it is all over has been a great weight lifted, and I was honestly happy as I walked across campus. I love you lots and lots. Give my love to Nanna.

Love,
Jenn

Wednesday seemed interminable. I still had difficulty moving, even though the lymph node surgery was healing. The much longer mastectomy incision simply hurt a lot. And, again, until allowed out of bed, I had to lie on my back, which made it ache. I counted the hours as I thought about how long it would take Bob to get back to Brussels. When he had not arrived by 2 p.m., I worried. What would I do if he had an accident? When one is feeling bad, things always look bleak. Finally, at about 4 p.m., he arrived and I immediately felt better. Becky also came by just in case Bob had not gotten back and Mother needed a ride home. And with her, she brought dinner. The food had become such a joke to all of us, and evening meals were particularly awful. Two pieces of dry bread and a mystery accompaniment. Never have meals tasted so wonderful as what Becky brought in thermoses and microwave containers every night for the rest of my stay in the hospital.

By Thursday I could move around. Although I had more pain, I felt livelier and ready to get on with things. I continued physical therapy and had very little difficulty in doing e-mail by myself. At lunch my roommate and I shared our high cholesterol tasteless meal. I discovered that Bridgette was a Brussels policewoman with the canine corps. We shared surgical stories, and she told me that in her police training she had learned that the most elite warriors among Amazon women voluntarily cut off their right breasts so that they could draw a bow and arrow better. We laughed that I would fit right in if only I were an Amazon archer. She told me she had undergone abdominal surgery, but it was not for cancer. I wondered if that were true. After all, we were in a cancer institute, and I knew that doctors were not always open with patients in this system. A young woman, Bridgette did physical exercises each day. She looked forward to going home on Saturday after a ten-day stay. Unlike her, I was raring to go and eager to get home by the weekend after only five days. This being my second stay in the hospital, I found Dr. Jaques' prediction coming true. I felt a bit bored.

During this week, the Belgian weather improved from the temperatures during my first stay, so I had more visitors. In addition to Mother coming every day, several visitors traveled from Mons and Brussels. Paddy brought greetings from the Mons Breast Cancer Support Group, which she had formed even though she herself did not have breast cancer. An informal group of British and American women, it provided a good source of sharing and healing. Mieke brought beautiful jonquils, a variety that her father, a botanist, had developed as a hybrid. A chaplain whom I did not know came from the military base with a kind word and prayer. The most significant visit, however, came from a classy, petite Belgian lady named Madame Carstairs.

I had read in Susan Love's book about a group called Reach to Recovery. Sponsored by the American Cancer Society, this group of breast cancer survivors visits breast cancer patients. They deliver a temporary prosthesis, talk to patients about caring for their affected arm after lymph node dissection, offer information about buying wigs and prostheses, and discuss other fears and questions. I had felt very sorry for myself not being in the United States to receive a Reach to Recovery visit. The Belgian social worker had visited one day and spoke only Flemish. All I understood was that she talked about a prosthesis and would come back another time. Even the literature was in French and Flemish. I could read some of it, but not to the level of detail that I needed. I worried about what I would do for a prosthesis. I had asked Mother to bring catalogues in the event I needed to order one from the States. But, by the time I had two operations, I had spent all my energy on treatment and never got around to choosing something to wear after the mastectomy.

To the rescue came Madame Carstairs. Without notice on Friday morning, in walked a lovely Belgian woman in a clinging sweater. Well-dressed and quite smart looking, she explained to me that she visited on behalf of *Vivre Comme Avant* (To Live As Before), the Belgian affiliate of Reach to Recovery. I got very teary-eyed and gushed out my gratitude. She explained that she also had had a mastectomy. As I looked at her form-fitting sweater, I would never have known any difference. What an inspiration! The doctors at Bordet would not permit the *Vivre Comme Avant* volunteers to demonstrate exercises to regain mobility, which was truly a shame, but she provided literature about wigs and prostheses. Most important, she made me a temporary prosthesis. She pinned it inside the bra I had worn to the hospital, making me ready to go out in public. She was my hero.

Dr. Hertens left on Friday for a medical congress in Paris, and she had explained that her assistants would remove the drains in her absence. If the drains could be removed, then I could be released on Saturday morning. Ashley would attend the Winter Formal on Saturday, so I wanted to be home. For months she had planned a party at our home before the dance. When I became ill, several of the other girls' mothers kindly offered to take over hosting the pre-dance party, and Ashley became quite upset. She didn't want anyone to usurp her position as the hostess. We had done all the shopping for her party the day before I returned to Bordet for the second surgery, and I knew that my mother would pull it off whether I arrived home or not. But I did so want to see the kids in all their finery.

Luckily, on Friday afternoon, the assistants removed the drains. I thought that this time I would be prepared, knowing the discomfort of removing the drains from the first surgery. Little did I know that this would be even worse because the incision was so much longer. It felt like my insides were coming right out with the drain.

Finally able to breathe again, I stammered, "*Je pense que je dit 'merci,' mais peut être non!*" ("I think that I say 'thank you,' but maybe not!") The two residents got a huge laugh out of that and commented that my French had certainly improved after two weeks in the hospital.

A ray of sunshine arrived that afternoon and brightened my day. Months before, Sarah had sent a package via a Belgian woman visiting a friend in Saint Petersburg, but it had never arrived. When the courier finally called, she learned I was in Bordet and she delivered the package to me there. When the nurse brought it in to me and I saw the package, it felt as though Sarah had walked into my room. I immediately perked up. Maybe it had been delayed for a reason, arriving at a time when I felt a bit low and particularly missed Sarah.

The one decision still awaiting us concerned the follow-on treatment I would receive. Dr. Hertens waited for test results showing the status of estrogen-receptors. If positive, then she would recommend tamoxifen and no chemotherapy. Dr. Jaques continued to say that because of my relatively young age, I should not be treated as a post-menopausal woman. All of this seemed very confusing.

Also confusing was that Dr. Hertens had so positively said that no cancer remained in my body; but in fact, no one could be sure of that, especially since I had one positive lymph node. I hated to dash the good spirits of my friends and family, but I needed to share the truth. It bothered me that everyone considered me completely out of the woods. I did not feel that way, nor did I feel strong and able to make these decisions alone.

The first help came from the wife of the U.S. Ambassador to Belgium, herself an ovarian cancer survivor. She recommended that I see Dr. Pincher, the head of oncology at Jules Bordet. She had helped Dr. Pincher both in the States and in Belgium with fundraising, and her own doctor had been Dr. Pincher's supervisor during a U.S.-based residency. I requested to talk to Dr. Pincher, but she was unavailable to see me during my hospitalization. She offered to meet me when I came to have the stitches removed the following week.

On Saturday morning, I heard the good news that I could go home. As I dressed, I blessed Madame Carstairs for helping me look more natural in front of Ashley's friends. Her party would be my "coming out" party.

The Roller Coaster Ride

Ashley's party was a success, and she looked lovely. Along with the two dozen high schoolers, there were a dozen moms who acted as chauffeurs, since driving age in Belgium is eighteen. We held a small adult gathering in the family room. While people knew I had been in the hospital, probably few realized that I had arrived home that afternoon. Everyone was kind, but no one wanted to talk about my surgery. I mean, what do you say to someone who has been diagnosed with cancer and is throwing a party? I wore the soft cotton prosthesis from Madame Carstairs over the bandages. I didn't look ravishing, but there were no visible signs of the surgery. As soon as they all left, I collapsed.

The next day I wrote to my e-mail support group:

January 26, 1997

Dear friends and family,

Today is Sunday. I was released from the Jules Bordet Cancer Institute yesterday. I got home in time to watch while my mother and Bob hosted about twenty of Ashley's friends for hors d'oeuvres prior to the Winter Formal. They were so cute, all dressed up to kill, enjoying shrimp cocktail and egg rolls, and sparkling grape juice in wine glasses. What a great coming-home present.

I'm so glad to be back home. I'm sore and very tired, but I feel both upbeat and whole. Next week I'll meet with the surgeon to get stitches out and with the oncologist to see about follow-on treatment. Because there was some lymph node involvement, it is assumed that there is some spread of cancer, and we will decide about next steps.

48

I've been thinking about the advantages of breast cancer:
- *two new pairs of Victoria's Secret pajamas*
- *a house full of flowers*
- *wonderful gifts of body cream, bath oils, and other assorted goodies for pampering oneself*
- *lots of meals brought in*
- *two weeks with my mother*
- *lots of time to read*
- *lots of phone calls from folks around the world*
- *seeing truly how much my husband and daughters love me*
- *seeing how competent my colleagues are who keep the business running smoothly without me*
- *knowing that I have friends and family like you who pray for me and send love and support. I feel quite covered by the prayers of my Jewish, Muslim, Catholic, and Protestant friends. I feel blessed and well cared for.*

Love,
Barbara

Despite the upbeat message, the next two weeks introduced me to the roller coaster of emotions that accompany cancer treatment. The first phase of treatment had seemed so clear: get the cancer out of the body. It may have taken two operations, but it presented a clear and actionable choice. Now, I seemed to be back in a limbo of uncertainty and decision-making.

Mother stayed with me for another week following my hospital release. Kind friends brought dinners and sent flowers and gifts. One of my very favorite gifts was a bronze cross that read *"Je suis avec vous"* (I am with you). It joined my table of symbols along with the red-hatted gnome and the photo collage of my family. My dear Belgian friend, Janine, brought wonderful homemade bouillon with a note that read:

I prepared this bouillon especially for you. Recipe: a lot of fresh vegetables for vitamins; a lot of love for your heart.

Her granddaughter, Alexandra, came along, and brought special pictures she had drawn to help me get well.

On January 31, just six days after I got out of the hospital, Jenn turned twenty-one. Before my diagnosis, we had planned a wonderful celebration in the States. Scheduled to be in Virginia on business, I would meet Jenn in northern Virginia. We had dinner plans on Friday night. On Saturday, our friend Linda would go with the two of us for a special personal shopping day for Jenn, and on Saturday night we had tickets for the Andrew Lloyd-Webber production at the National Theater, *Whistle Down the Wind*. Of course, I could not go to Virginia, so we decided that Bob would fly in just for the weekend to take Jenn to dinner and the theater. Linda would take her for the shopping trip.

Mother hoped to return to Florida in time for my stepfather's birthday on February 2, so it seemed to make sense that she would fly out with Bob on January 31. That made it easier for them both to travel to the airport in Brussels. I hadn't driven yet, so we planned that Bob would take me to Brussels on January 30 to have my stitches removed. I booked an appointment on the same afternoon with Dr. Pincher, the chief of oncology. Early in the week, we received a call asking if we could come to the clinic on Wednesday, a day earlier, because Dr. Pincher was not available on Thursday. I asked if Dr. Hertens had been consulted to see if my stitches could be removed on Wednesday and they said that would be suitable.

On Wednesday morning, I had my first physical therapy session with Marie Joris at the military clinic in Mons. She had previously worked at Jules Bordet and was wonderfully attuned to the needs of cancer patients. Still heavily bandaged, I could not do too much, but she began lymph massage on my affected arm. Her gentle touch and soothing manner were to become a positive part of my recovery. The rest of the day, however, did not turn out well.

In the afternoon, we drove to the cancer institute in Brussels. The bus drivers all across Belgium were on strike and had converged on the city. Buses were parked all over the place and streets were closed. Protestors blocked the best route to the hospital. We eventually found the hospital, arriving a few minutes late. Apparently, the assistants who changed my appointment day had not confirmed with the doctors. Dr. Hertens said it was too early to take out the stitches. She checked the incision, drained off lymph fluid, and bandaged me back up.

We were startled to find that despite the appointment change, Dr. Pincher still would not see us. Without any explanation, she referred us to someone else. At that point, Bob became angry. Dr. Hertens called Dr.

Pincher who remained unwilling to accommodate us, but agreed to a telephone consult the next day. We met instead with Dr. Kenton, an oncologist from Luxembourg who spoke excellent English. He explained the two chemotherapy protocols and confirmed that Jules Bordet did not think I should have chemotherapy.

"Why is there a difference in the recommendation between the Belgians and the Americans?" I asked.

"The Americans are too aggressive," he casually responded with a shrug.

He gave me some good information, allowing me to ask better questions, but his bedside manner left a lot to be desired. We left Bordet feeling discouraged.

The decision about follow-on treatment proved difficult. Bordet recommended only tamoxifen—an endocrine-based chemo taken by pill—for five years. The immediate side effects were not as severe as with traditional chemo. The more difficult decision was whether to opt for traditional chemo in addition to the tamoxifen. The immediate side effects would be more severe (hair loss, vomiting, nausea, fatigue) and depending on the type of chemo, it would take either three or six months. No one would say how much or if it would improve the odds against recurrence. Tamoxifen seemed to be the easy choice, but I did not want to take the easy short-term choice at the expense of long-term health. I felt stuck and alone on this decision.

Adding to my loneliness, Mother and Bob left very early on Friday morning for flights back to the States. Ashley traveled to Germany to cheer at a basketball game, leaving me very much alone for the first time. I managed with some difficulty to wash my hair and got myself to physical therapy in the afternoon. On my first attempt to drive, I found that I could not spin the wheel to turn and I had trouble looking hard left at a difficult intersection. The physical therapy lymph massage was nice, but the stretching hurt even at the gentle angle required because of the stitches.

Dr. Pincher had scheduled a telephone appointment for 10:15 on Friday, but she never called. When I tried to reach her, her assistant said she was not in. I mentioned this to Janine, who was furious. She called her friend, the Director at Jules Bordet, and insisted that Dr. Pincher call me, but I still did not hear from her.

I felt very sorry for myself, missing Jenn's twenty-first birthday. I called and woke her up to sing happy birthday, barely able to sing through the

51

tears. Later, Nancy arrived with dinner and movies for the evening. It became a comedy of errors when Nancy accidentally tripped the duress alarm and the police called to see if we had an emergency.

"I am calling to see if you are under duress," the Belgian voice asked. "Please give me the proper code."

"Code? I have no idea what is the code!" I responded, feeling like an idiot. Surely Bob must have told me the code word when the system had been activated more than a year earlier, but it escaped me at this point.

"If you do not provide the code, we assume you are under duress. We will send the local police to surround the house. You must come out of the house with identification and your hands in the air."

I felt plenty of duress, but not from either an intruder or the police. Somehow I persuaded my kind protector that emergency actions were unnecessary.

"We are just two flaky women who pushed the wrong button," I said, wondering if he knew the meaning of "flaky." Thank goodness that ended the excitement for the evening.

On Saturday morning, I drove to the health clinic to meet Chris Georgantopoulos who would take out my stitches. It seemed to take him forever, and I lay on the table with tears in my eyes—not from the discomfort, but from thinking how much I would rather be in Virginia celebrating Jenn's birthday. He kindly asked if I wanted to talk, but I just shook my head, no.

February 1

To Mother, Bob, Kennon:

I've just returned from getting the stitches out-twenty-three of them. The incision is lots longer than I thought. It goes diagonally from the breast bone up to the middle of my arm pit. Dr. Georgantopoulos said the stitches were very tight—meaning a better cosmetic effect but very difficult to take out. He really struggled. Without all the bandages, my skin is much more sensitive. I had worn one of Bob's shirts to the clinic, but came home with an aqua cotton doctor's tunic on. Right now I have on the nice, soft, pajama top KP sent. And I have finally been able to wash under my arm for the first time in twenty-six days. What a relief.

Last night at about 11:45, I received a call from Dr. Frank Ward at Walter Reed. He treated Max and he is also the consulting oncologist to the Surgeon General. He was very kind and took lots of information. He recommended chemo and said if I were at Walter Reed, I would be part of a new protocol testing the effects on post-menopausal women. Dr. G had gotten the same answer from his consultants in Ottawa, so I guess I will try to start chemo in the next two weeks.

I'm feeling pretty down today. I'm really missing Bob and all the birthday celebrations, but I'm so glad Bob and Jenn are together. It's also looking like I won't be going anywhere for a while with the chemo. Because the recommended protocol is highly toxic, Dr. Ward said I shouldn't fly.

I read last night that the survival rate for women with breast cancer is higher when they are married and have supportive families. I'm blessed with the support of all of you. I love you very much.

Barbara

Ashley returned from her game in Germany not feeling well. She felt tired and sick, I felt tired and depressed, and that did not make for a good combination. We were both short-tempered with each other. However, that provided a catalyst to discover what was bothering both of us. As we turned our grousing into good conversation, we had a wonderful talk and cry together, and it helped us both.

She admitted that she did not want to talk about the cancer because she wanted everything to be "normal." She hadn't told any of her friends about the cancer, and when people would ask her how I was, she would happily respond, "Fine." I explained to her that her response was confusing and didn't allow others to help her.

"Why don't Jenn and Sarah have to be here?" she raged. "Why am I the only one who gets stuck here dealing with you being sick! It's not fair!"

"Jenn and Sarah are actually angry that they are not here," I reminded her. "Maybe if you talk to them and e-mail them to share the experience, it would help all three of you. Talking to your friends could also help."

Ashley admitted she had broken down in school the week before and reacted angrily to her U.S. History teacher who gave her a hard time about making up work she had missed during the week of Model UN in The Hague. Ashley ended up hiccuping and crying so hard that the teacher sent her out of the room.

"Mom, I really don't want you to have chemo," she said. "I don't want people to know you're bald!"

Saying all that out loud released the dam and started Ashley's healing. She became a great companion and support.

On Sunday, I called Dr. Jim Hines, a friend of Kennon and Howard and himself a cancer survivor. Jim had been the Chief of Surgery at Northwestern University Hospital in Chicago. He had earlier told Kennon that he favored mastectomy over lumpectomy. He believed that if cancer grew in tissue, then you removed the "field" in which it grew, not just the cancer itself. I wished I had followed his advice on my first surgery. Jim had consulted with Howard on his surgery and insisted that they remove additional sections of the colon on either side of Howard's tumor. A year after Howard's surgery, Jim died of complications from hepatitis that he had contracted as an Army doctor during the Korean War. What a loss—he was a fantastic advisor to me when I desperately needed guidance.

February 1, 1997

Hi KP,

I just talked to both Jim and Hollis. I didn't realize that she had a mastectomy twenty years ago. Both were so delightful and encouraging. Jim made the explanation quite simple. The chemo and the tamoxifen do different things. The chemo kills cancer that's there. The tamoxifen prevents the spread but doesn't kill it. He said to him the chemo is like buying insurance. You can't go back and buy it after you've already had an accident, robbery, or died. Makes sense to me. Thanks for setting up the phone call.

Love,
Barbara

Becky and Randy visited on Sunday. With the stitches out and bandages off, I could not tolerate fabric next to my skin. My whole chest turned yellow with bruising. Randy didn't seem to mind that I entertained them in a pajama top, clearly lop-sided underneath, and I felt too tired and sore to care. Becky brought about a dozen shirts that I could wear, all of them soft and buttoning up the front so I could get my arm into them. Getting things over my head was nearly impossible, and I needed something loose to wear to physical therapy.

Marie Joris was the kindest, gentlest physical therapist I could imagine. Now that the stitches were out, we really went to work. Daily, she massaged the scar so it would not form too much scar tissue inside. That kind of intimate touching could have been awkward, but Marie was gentle and empathetic. She massaged the whole length of my arm to help with lymph drainage, and she stretched my arm to increase range of motion. After two operations and limited mobility for almost a month, I could not reach up-ward much at all, and the stretching was very painful. She could determine the amount of pain by watching my feet. As the pain grew worse, my feet would rise off the table. Not breathing, I couldn't tell her how much it hurt.

Bob returned home on Monday after the birthday celebration in Vir-ginia. Having made it through the weekend alone, begun driving again, gotten the stitches out, and weathered the emotional talk with Ashley, I now just gave in to weakness.

February 3, 1997

Hi, Mom and KP,

Yesterday was a bad day. I had to drive three times between 7 a.m. and 1 p.m. for Ashley and physical therapy. I was just ex-hausted, and after Bob got home, I didn't have to be strong any-more. I couldn't stop crying all day. Finally, about 1 a.m. I was so drained I fell asleep.

Hopefully I'll talk to the oncologist tomorrow. It has been a battle to get to talk to her—and that drains me, too. The language diffi-culty and some very unhelpful secretaries at Jules Bordet seem to conspire against our connecting.

My physical therapy has been increased to every day. I guess with the two surgeries, my arm was dormant for so long that it is harder to stretch it out. It is very painful.

We have a big dinner tonight to farewell Bob's boss and wife, but I think I won't go. The incision is so uncomfortable that I don't tolerate clothes very well. Your pajama top is the best thing I can wear, and I doubt that would look very good at a fancy dinner.

Mother responded:

So sorry you didn't feel up to going to the dinner. The sooner you can get to doing things the better it will be for your morale. After your father died, a friend told me that I must make myself go out and do things, that once I got there I would forget my problems for a while and enjoy myself. I didn't really believe her but when I tried it she was right. I realize right now that you are hurting physically and mentally. But please try to get back to normal as soon as possible. You will profit from it in the long run.

My cousin, an Episcopal priest who had performed the marriage ceremony for Bob and me twenty-seven years before, sent "a love message across the miles" that also reminded me of Bob's suffering in all of this.

February 3, 1997

Dear Barbara,

Judy and I just got word from your mother about you. We both want you to know that you are in our prayers and that we are thinking of you and Bob. You will be hearing from many people, I am sure, who have been through cancer. People will show up from the most distant of places to tell you about their bouts with breast cancer. What you will find out in all of this, I suspect, is that there is a huge, absolutely gigantic, network of people around the world that has experienced breast cancer. That is a good thing to know and is comforting in many ways as you go through all of this and need to draw strength and insight from other folks. It is a blessing.

At the same time, no one can know what you know about what you are going through because no one is you. You will have your own feelings and thoughts that no one will be able to read or understand no matter how sensitive or knowledgeable they may be. I am sure that you will be spending time dealing with people you care about over the gap between what they are able to know with you and what is out of their reach.

As you know, Judy went through a lumpectomy about fifteen years ago and a mastectomy just before we left Raleigh three years ago. Being an oncology nurse herself, it was both a blessing and a curse in my opinion. To suffer an illness in your own specialty is a difficult experience, and yet, I do believe that all of the people she had worked with, and continued to work with, who had cancer were a support to her. Cancer patients, by her own definition, are a special kind of people. Because of the closeness and empathy she felt with them, she was able to transfer a great deal of that contact into her own struggle.

I know that it was most difficult to see her go through this. It brought me close to the power of death. I see a great deal of death in people's lives in the work I do. I live with death as a constant companion but it is always thee and thee and not me. Judy as the ill person brought the thee home to me. It was a fearful time, a time when I once again came up against the anticipation of her death and mine as well. The images of separation were strong and terrifying. Just the thought of cancer in her and the possibility that she might be gone made me very sad. I don't know where Bob is with all of this but I suspect he will also bump up against some of the same kind of emotions. They are very normal and talking all of that out will be crucial.

I love you and Judy joins me in that love. We want to stay in touch and be here prayerfully in any way that we can. Love to you, Bob. Know that there are lots of men who have walked this path with their wives and who have drawn strength from them and one another.

Love,
Jim

To Have or Have Not— The Chemotherapy Dilemma

It required an enormous amount of energy to fight the Belgian medical system and to try to connect with Dr. Pincher, the chief of oncology at Jules Bordet. It depressed and tired me. For two weeks, I had continually called her and she never returned my calls. Bouncing back from surgery proved harder this time, probably because of having general anesthesia twice within two weeks. And the three weeks of immobility for my arm made it very stiff and painful.

Marie, my physical therapist, finally reached Dr. Pincher for me. Marie knew Dr. Pincher from her days at Bordet, and she worked through the secretaries to get Dr. Pincher on the phone. Even after being personally called by the U.S. Ambassador's wife, and after Belgian friends Janine and Paul had both called the Director of Bordet as well as Dr. Pincher's secretary, she had never called me back. She acted quite haughty, saying I had failed to keep an appointment with her. I reminded her that she had changed an appointment with me and then refused to see me. She had failed to keep a telephone appointment that she arranged, and then never returned my calls.

"You're talking to the wrong doctors," she nearly screamed at me. "They give you bad advice, and I will not give you chemotherapy. The Tumor Board has closed your case."

I decided immediately that I could not be treated by a doctor like that. It was not worth arguing with her. Even Dr. Kenton, who had little bed-side manner, appeared to be more forthcoming and kinder. I made an appointment to see him the following week. That night I had a terrible dream about chemo and doctors who would not talk to me. Kennon, a Jungian analyst who works with dreams in her clinical practice, wrote:

Bad dreams have an important purpose. They are trying to get your attention and make you conscious of something you must know. You have made the right decision about changing oncologists. A doctor whose attitude is wrong, no matter how good he or she is technically, cannot heal. The relationship between the patient and the doctor is essential to make the chemo work. You must be able to feel that the oncologist is right there with you and available for all your questions and fears.

Jim Hines would be out of his mind if he heard your story about this doctor. He has no patience for doctors who cannot "hold" the patient through the experience. If the male doctor can do this, go with him.

Last night I had a dream about my left breast being cut into, a long incision right through it. I awoke thinking about you and feeling a little bit of what you must be feeling. You will need a lot of emotional support as you go into the chemo. Try to go very slowly, do not think ahead but only of this moment and above all put your energy into your own healing.

By the end of the week, I felt better. Decisions were made and friends sent love and encouragement. With so much love coming to me, I couldn't stay down for too long, so I shared the encouragement with my support group.

February 9

Hi All,

It is Sunday and the sun is out, and I'm feeling better. Ashley got off yesterday on her ski trip. I can imagine her schussing down the slopes in Garmisch, and I wish we were there. We are calling Sarah later tonight to find out how she is.

My Canadian doctor called me yesterday from the States. He is at a conference in Virginia Beach. He got through to the head of breast cancer research at the National Cancer Institute, and he called to let me know the conversation. That oncologist also agrees that I should have the chemo, and even advised on what type. I'll call the Belgian oncologist tomorrow to alert him I'm coming on Wednesday. If he

agrees to go with the recommended regimen, I will definitely lose my
hair, so Bob and I will go wig shopping on Wednesday.

Love,

Barbara

When we talked to Sarah, we found her in a much better state, and that helped me too. Her wonderful Russian mother, Irina, was the director of the medical laboratory at a Russian Army hospital. She knew a lot about breast cancer and spent time with Sarah talking about the treatment and the advantages of early detection. I had also sent Lillie Shockney's book, *Joining the Club*, to Sarah. I told Sarah it would help her know what was happening at home. She read it immediately and wrote down all the questions she wanted to ask me. She asked excellent questions, things she probably would not have had the nerve to ask were she on the spot.

During our telephone conversation, Sarah said that she had two important things to tell me.

"Mom, you used your breasts to nurse all three of us, and you don't need them any more. And you are successful in business and in life because of your mind, not your body. So, you're the same person and you'll still be successful and whole even without a breast."

I was in tears as she finished this sermon. What a wonderful reversal to have my eighteen-year-old daughter telling her forty-eight-year-old mother how to get on with life.

Kennon had sent a large box of tapes, books, and assorted things to help me through the process. As I felt better, I delved into those things and also began taking a regimen of royal jelly, recommended by a French friend, Danielle. I had never paid a lot of attention to natural healing, but my confronting cancer opened a world of alternatives. I felt scared enough and determined enough that I would try anything that was not harmful to my health. My friend Mieke had told me about the writings of Andrew Weil, and I read his *Spontaneous Healing* with interest. There seemed to be many ways to kick this disease that would supplement and help the traditional methods of surgery and chemotherapy.

Mieke also introduced me to her friend Christine, who was suffering from a recurrence of breast cancer, metastasized to her liver. Although Christine and I only met twice in the months ahead, she provided wise counsel by e-mail and telephone, and she helped me get beyond my anger at Dr. Pincher. After all, anger drains energy, and I needed all the energy I had to fight the disease and get through the chemotherapy.

60

Part Two
Support

Separately,
We are as
Fragile as reeds
And as easily
Broken.

But together,
We are as strong
As reeds tied
In a bundle.

Inspired by Jewish Writings

Some Kind of Hair Day

Having made the decision to have chemotherapy, I wanted to start it immediately. The treatment would last for three months, leaving only a month to prepare for our expected trans-Atlantic move back to the States. The idea exhausted me.

We traveled to Jules Bordet on February 12 and met Mieke's friend Christine after her morning appointment. She accompanied us to the wig shop, but we were dismayed to find it closed over the lunch hour. Christine advised us on how to choose a wig if we returned after the appointment with Dr. Kenton.

When we met with Dr. Kenton, we found him very willing to accommodate our request for chemotherapy. He concurred with the American oncologists who recommended the three-month regimen of Adriamycin and cyclophosphamide. Dr. Kenton's casual attitude proved helpful in persuading him to treat me with chemotherapy, given his director's refusal. However, it also meant that he did not "hold" me through the treatment as Jim Hines had said a good oncologist must do. For that level of care, I depended on Chris Georgantopoulos, even though he was not an oncologist.

I had also consulted by phone with Dr. Louis Diehl, chief of oncology at the Walter Reed Army Medical Center. He helpfully outlined the various options, confirming that I must have chemotherapy with even one positive lymph node. As he explained it, no positive lymph nodes meant a 75 percent chance that the cancer had not spread. One to four positive lymph nodes translated to a fifty-fifty chance that the cancer had spread. And more than four positive lymph nodes meant a 90 percent chance of spread to other parts of the body, most likely the liver, lungs, bones, or brain.

Dr. Diehl referred me to his oncology nurse, Jane Shotkin. My telephone and e-mail relationship with Jane became very valuable to me. She prepared me for a myriad of things that no one else mentioned to me. For instance, immediately after the treatment, my urine would be red. No one else ever told me that, and I can imagine how terrified I would have been had I not known it. Jane talked a lot about hair loss, buying a prosthesis, and the side effects of chemo and how to avoid them. She encouraged me to use mouth-wash to avoid mouth sores, to drink a lot of water, and to walk a lot. She said I would gain weight, which, unfortunately, I did. If my temperature ever reached 100.4°, I knew to go to the emergency room and tell the doctors I was taking chemo and to start me immediately on antibiotics. I should not have dental care during chemotherapy. And if my blood counts were too low between treatments, I should delay the next treatment.

Adriamycin can be quite toxic to the heart. In fact, Susan Love reports that some children treated with Adriamycin for childhood cancers later experienced heart failure. Therefore, the treatment was limited to four three-week cycles. Before beginning chemo, I needed a MUGA (multi-gated acquisition) scan of my heart to determine its health and potential effects of the caustic Adriamycin. Therefore, I could not start the chemo that day. Dr. Kenton scheduled the MUGA scan for the next day. If the results came back showing a strong heart, then I could start chemo immediately.

Bob and I returned to the wig store, finding it open. The woman in the shop spoke only Flemish, so we were lost in communicating. All the wigs were synthetic and the selection seemed limited. I still had a full head of hair, making it difficult to try wigs on. I felt pressured to buy something so I would have a wig when I needed it. Finally, I chose the lesser of the evils—a blonde wig about the length of my own hair but with lots of hair in it. It matched the color of the highlighted part of my hair and had fat curls. I hoped that I would learn to style it, but at the moment I felt like I had a bowl of blonde curls perched on top of my head.

I simply could not stand to try any more styles on. The small shop, which featured a huge display window, made me feel claustrophobic, as though I were in a fish tank. I just wanted to get out of there.

When I asked Bob to pay for the blonde bombshell, I was astounded to see the price of over $300. Did wigs really cost that much? Bob bought me a red terrycloth turban as my valentine gift, and it would become my favorite head covering.

All this activity exhausted me. For days it seemed as though all I had done was get up, bathe, make the bed, go to physical therapy, take a nap, and put something on the table for dinner, so I could go back to bed. That night I didn't sleep very well with the anticipation of starting the poison the next morning.

February 13

To family:

Bob and I spent all day at Jules Bordet. I had a baseline blood test to look at white count and platelets. Then I had a MUGA scan of my heart. It took over an hour. First I drank some yucky radioactive stuff. Then they injected me with more radioactive stuff, and I lay on a very narrow table for forty minutes while a big camera (shaped like an enormous frisbee) rotated around my body taking pictures. Then they injected more radioactive stuff, waited fifteen minutes, injected MORE radioactive stuff and the frisbee camera took pictures from two angles above my heart. I was not allowed to talk during this session as talking speeds up the heart rate.

We had time for a quick lunch, then met again with the oncologist. The MUGA scan results were fine and blood counts in the normal range, so we went for the first chemo treatment. Nothing's easy-again, we first had to settle an argument with the admissions folks about taking our insurance. Finally, someone who spoke English came to help us, apologized for the bad humor of the woman who refused our insurance papers, and escorted us to the "hopital du jour" for outpatient treatment. The chemo itself took less than an hour. Five bags of stuff—first fluid to lubricate the system, then anti-nausea medication, then the worst toxin (Adriamycin) which is red. If it touches your skin, you get bad burns, and it causes you to pee red for the first few days. Then a clear bag of the other poison (cyclophosphamide), followed by another bag of fluid to clean the veins. Including the MUGA scan, blood tests and the chemotherapy, I should have received five "sticks" today—needles of some sort. But, my veins have never been cooperative, and I can no longer receive any kind of needles in my arm on the mastectomy side. So, I now have closer to nine bruises from needles, rather than just five.

They have given me anti-nausea pills to take for the next three mornings. They have told me to use mouthwash several times every day to help prevent sores in my mouth. And they said my hair will fall out suddenly about day fifteen.

Love,
Barbara

The next morning, Valentine's Day, I updated my support group:

February 14

To Support Group:
Happy Valentine's Day to all—seems like I have a long list of "sweethearts" this year, and I thank you again for all your love. First chemo session was yesterday and the anti-nausea drugs are working. The chemo is red and Bob gave me a red turban—seems fitting for the day.

Love,
Barbara

My e-mail support group rallied around as I started the process of chemotherapy. Business colleagues were beginning to hear about my situation, and associates from my professional trade association joined the group of well-wishers, prayer warriors, and morale lifters. I discovered, too, that there is a special sorority of women who have gone through the treatment for breast cancer. As Lillie Shockney described in her book, we had "joined the club." That meant that I even heard from friends of friends who were part of the club. One such person, whom I never met, provided helpful advice.

February 12, 1997

Dear Barbara,
You don't know me. I've worked with Jack for entirely too many years, and he shared your health situation with me. I completed my chemo for breast cancer three years and six months ago. I'm one of those markers you can use to say to yourself: this too will pass. Not to minimize it, because chemo is a truly awesome experience.
I suggest you do more than the wig. Pay a visit to someone who can help you learn to apply eyebrows and eyeliner—it's not just the hair on your head that disappears. I found that a) the hair loss

affected my spirits more than the actual chemo, and b) I felt very superficial because of that. My oncologist's clinical nurse specialist was helpful: she reminded me that it wasn't my vanity alone. Every time I looked in the mirror at that bald lady, I saw a woman with cancer. She was right. Keep that in mind. Also invest in trés chic headcoverings of multiple styles (wraps, turbans, cloche hats), including something you can wear to bed at night. My mother made me some flannel Amish-style bonnets that tied under my chin. I never had a cold head—or appeared bald to my family.

What is it, I wondered, that makes it so difficult for a woman to lose her hair? Kennon wrote:

> *February 14, 1997*
>
> *How are you feeling about losing your hair? I realized that that would be more upsetting to me than losing a breast. Isn't that interesting? After I had that dream about my breast being cut in half, lengthwise, I started putting myself in your place and aside from not wanting cancer, surgery, pain, physical therapy, poisons in my system (have I left anything out?), what I knew would be hard for me was losing my hair. And I don't even have great hair. I have thin, oily, mouse-colored strands that have caused me anguish much of my life because of "bad hair days." So what's my problem? Well, I discovered my sense of femininity is connected with my hair more than with my breasts. Maybe a wig is the answer and that's what I need to discover.*

I responded to Kennon:

> *Everything I have read says losing your hair is the most traumatic part of the treatment, even though you know your hair will grow back. I think I'm coping quite well with the lost breast. Although, it's kind of funny. I've always thought I was pretty flat-chested. Now I know what really flat-chested is, and I realize I had more than I thought. One side of my chest is absolutely concave. Nonetheless, I'm still wandering around in men's undershirts and not too worried about it. If I go out, I wear another shirt on top, but not always buttoned.*

I've just ordered two more wigs from a catalog. I'm not sure I'm happy with the $300 wig I just bought. I worked with it a little more today and felt a little happier, but I find it hard to style. And it is very blonde so I don't feel like me. Of course, that's the color I chose so I have no one to blame but myself. I was advised to get synthetic wigs because they're easier to care for. I'm not sure that's a good idea either. The oncology nurse says I will lose all my hair by day fifteen and that's now less than two weeks away.

A couple people have suggested getting an assortment of wigs in different styles and colors. But my reaction to the very blonde wig seems to be evidence that I want something more like my own hair. The ones I ordered are both frosted.

I have taken a nap this afternoon, but I still feel amazingly good. We are going to Brussels tonight to the sixtieth birthday celebration of our Danish friend. They had planned the date specifically around our availability, and I'm glad we won't let them down. If I get too tired, we'll just leave early. Now I'd better go find some clothes to wear. It will be my first venture out in dress clothes.

Many folks offered suggestions for dealing with the hair loss: turbans, scarves, hats, or even going bald. Ashley thought I should shave my head before my hair fell out. Jennifer concurred, saying that shaving my head would put me in control. While I didn't go to the extreme of shaving my head, I decided that Ashley had a great idea and that, as Jennifer said, the issue of control was important to me. So, I had a hairdresser come to the house and cut my hair into a very short pixie. I sent out an e-mail titled "Shorn!"

February 19

Dear friends and family,

My support group list (you) continues to grow, and your messages make me feel so much better. Please stay in touch. Today is day seven of the first chemo cycle. I have chemo on day one and wait three weeks for the next three-week cycle. This continues for four rounds. My counts should start dropping tomorrow and the "danger" period is between days eight and fifteen. By day fifteen, my hair should be history. I decided to help the process along in order to feel more in control. Today a hairdresser came to the house and cut my hair short. I have had it frosted for so many years that I didn't realize that it is really brown. What a shock. I called Bob to warn him that the strange woman in the house is really me. Otherwise, he might not know what to do when he comes home. A dear friend brought me an American Cancer Society catalog full of hats, and I think I'll order some. I'm still struggling with the blonde curly wig— it just isn't me. Other friends have told me I should follow Princess Caroline's lead (she has lost her hair from alopoecia) and wear lovely Hermés scarves. I'm afraid all that I have in common with the Princess is the scarves—not the gorgeous looks to go with them.

I've felt amazingly okay since the chemo. No nausea, just occasional queasiness. Over the weekend I was exhausted and spent most of the time in bed, but I feel better this week. Next week I'll have to be careful since I'll be susceptible to infection.

The physical therapy continues daily and I am regaining mobility in my arm and use of the chest muscles. No signs of swelling from the lymph node dissection—all good news.

I'm told the hardest psychological part is losing my hair. I'm hoping to make it through the next three months gracefully, if bald. Haven't come up with a list of advantages to being bald, as I did for the top ten reasons to have breast cancer. Maybe you can help me out.

My support group was quick to return a huge list of positives for losing your hair.

If you think your hair is more important than your brains, it probably is....

My number one reason for going bald is—no bad hair days.

When some people lose their hair, it comes in curly. After spending hundreds of dollars on perms, if I could be guaranteed curly hair, I'd consider the hat/scarf thing for a few months. Wouldn't it be great if your hair came in curly and frosted? Think of the time saved. If the blond curly thing isn't working, would you like me to pick up one of the black headdresses used for Japanese theater when I am in Japan next month?

I wanted to pass on a practical advantage to being shorn—as someone with lots of experience. You can dry your hair (or head) with a wash cloth in one pass. It will add at least ten minutes to your day.

Thank goodness you do not have more in common with HRH Princess Caroline...and without a flutter of my eyelashes, I pronounce thee Queen....it's probably all right to be a princess...but I think you are a fine queen. In seriousness, we have a friend at home who turned to scarves almost entirely...turbans for dressier occasions, and bandana type for everyday and at-home wear. Very smart...very chic...very queenly. Whatever you choose will suit all of us who love you. Think that a year or so ago Calvin Klein made "bandana" pattern scarves in pastels...delicious colors. But, in my opinion, a good old red bandana like the farmers use should be a part of every girl's wardrobe.

You are lovely, even as a marine. Princess Caroline can't hold a candle to you.

Well, I have to tell you that Sinead O'Connor and Sigourney Weaver have always made MY heart go pitty-pat. It's the in thing. You're on the cutting edge of style.

You are looking for something good to be said about being bald— no more bad hair days for a while.

One positive thing I can think of about being bald is not having to figure out what color your hair will be when the beauticians get through with it. Up here in Connecticut, they seem to know how to make mine yellow or orange but nothing else. I've decided to take over the process myself. I figure I can ruin it for a lot less money. Hey, that's another thing. You'll save money for a while.

You could now be a "stunt double" for Telly Savalas, but a better idea is now you don't have to spend as much time "doing" your hair.

Gutsy lady to shear your hair first. Let's see...here are a few for your new top ten to add to what I'm sure others will send: 1) Scalp dries quicker than hair, 2) Simplifies getting dressed and "done up," 3) Good for circulation, 4) Closer to heaven—if heaven is up, that is, 5) Clears the path for the seventh chakra (at the crown of your head).

Advantages of no hair—think of all the extra time you will have each day not having to wash and fool with hair. Think of how much more you can accomplish in three months—or just have more time to rest and relax.

Tasteless Comment # 32—Hair today, gone tomorrow.

Okay so I may not be the funniest person alive, but let me see what I can do...
10. Save time washing hair
9. Save money on shampoo
8. No need to schedule appointments at the beauty parlor
7. Save tons of money (no more highlighting, cutting)
6. Save on your electricity bill (no hair dryer or curling iron)
5. No more wind-blown hair or tangles to deal with
4. No need to worry about all that gray
3. No need to worry about the weather's effect on your hair (humidity, rain)
2. Save on hair spray
1. No more "bad hair days"

No more perms or chemical processing, no more having to purchase hair products, no risk of head lice, and no bad hair days.

One of the advantages of being bald is that immediately you have a new look. I remember a strikingly beautiful bald woman in the first Star Trek film.
Another advantage is that you immediately move to a low maintenance status. Less time showering, drying, setting hair.

Hmmm...why be bald...well, take it from experience

(mine)...after the shower you can dry your hair real quick...save on hair goo...beards look better on bald men (sorry, no help there)...less hair in the drain...you can look like what's her name...that Irish gal...Sinead O'Connor something like that...but you do have something important going for you...it will grow back without expensive Chinese magic herbs.

Here are a few more pluses for baldness, our topic for conversation yesterday morning over coffee:
- *easier to spot if lost at sea, due to reflection*
- *advantage in competition, due to less wind resistance in bobsled race*
- *if caught by guests as you're running from the bathroom naked, simply freeze to be taken as a mannequin*
- *savings on hairspray, shampoo, conditioner, and curling devices, not to mention electricity in blow-drying your hair*
- *easier to camouflage in a truckful of melons if crossing a border illegally (my favorite)*

Advantages of being BALD. Let's see.......
save money on hair brushes
save the ozone layer because no hair spray
easier for satellites to detect you because of the reflective light
you can get a job as a cone-head on Saturday Night Live
Will save on Drano

My support group's creativity kept me laughing. The funniest stories about wigs came from Cindy.

Bald seems to be beautiful these days...Demi Moore, as an example.
As for your list, I've always heard that your hair will be much nicer when it grows back. You can verify that for me.
And as for wigs, they are hot and scratchy. I have always had very fine, thin hair, and have always envied those with thick curly locks. When I was a young girl of twenty-one-ish, those Eva Gabor wigs were in fashion. I had several styles, colors, and lengths. No

one ever saw my hair. But wigs do have drawbacks; the following stories are true.

1. I was standing at a check-out line in a Kmart type store in Denver, Colorado, with a particularly cute short, blond, frosted, shag wig on and my infant daughter (about six months old) in my arms, when suddenly, she pulled the wig off and threw it on the floor behind my shopping cart. Britt laughed....and I wanted to crawl away.

2. Having not learned to appreciate what God had given me, but now wearing a cute brown dutch-boy, I was riding in a bumper car in Germany at one of their many fests. If you've ever watched the Germans, they don't bump, but rather drive around in a nice circle. Well, I didn't know that, so I got in my car (the first time I'd ever—and last—been in bumpercars) and began bumping people. Everyone ganged up on me, I became the bumpee. I received one extremely vicious bump that sent my dutch-boy flying. It got caught under my car. By the time I retrieved it, it was no longer cute. Shortly thereafter, I gave up on wigs.

A thoughtful response came from Anne:

I think you are right that the loss of hair is the most difficult thing for most people—which, considering the nature of cancer and the issues one deals with in grappling with the illness, tells you something about the persistence of vanity in human nature. Most people find wigs hot and itchy. Hats may be the best bet. A friend had a great collection of baseball caps, including one with sequins for evenings. I will keep my eyes peeled for appropriate specimens.

Anne kept her promise. She sent a great sequined baseball cap, a copy of Bernie Siegal's *Love, Medicine and Miracles*, and Christine Clifford's *Not Now...I'm Having a No Hair Day.* In prose and cartoons, it told of Christine's battle with cancer and chemo and truly added humor into what was otherwise a difficult situation.

Why is hair loss so difficult? Kennon suggested that being bald allows one to see oneself in a way not often possible. That must bring a consciousness about one's self that others simply don't have. Perhaps it is that the persona is gone and we are more directly in touch with ourselves. There is nothing to hide behind. She asked me to tell her what the experience would be like, and she wondered if I would have hair in my dreams during this time.

As the fifteenth day got closer, I dreaded the hair loss. But it was totally out of my control. As my friend Roy suggested:

I know it has not been easy for you nor the family, but press on.
I don't think wearing a wig will detract, so just offer it up.

And since I had no choice, that's exactly what I did.

Nothing's Easy

The first week after my initial chemotherapy treatment seemed so uneventful that it took me by surprise on day nine of the cycle when I became terribly ill. Bob had scheduled meetings in The Hague, and I insisted that he go. I must be a slow learner, not remembering that I wished he had stayed behind on the trip to England during my second surgery. Chris Georgantopoulos proved his care, concern, and ability to "hold" the patient through treatment by coming to the house. I told him how to get in the back door and where he would find me, and he was as gentle and helpful as anyone could be. My friend Nancy and Bob's assistant, Liz, both checked on me during the day.

My e-mail message the next day was entitled "What a way to lose ten pounds."

February 22, 1997

Good morning. It is Saturday, and I think I'll live. (You know, suddenly, that takes on more meaning.) Yesterday was dreadful and scary. I woke up at 3:30 a.m. feeling awful. By 4:15, I was vomiting and then the diarrhea started for the next nine hours. Bob was being picked up at 6:30 to go to The Hague (Netherlands) for meetings. He said he didn't think he should leave me. Like an idiot, I told him he should go and I'd call for help if I needed it. But, of course, after he left I wished he were still here. I finally reached my Canadian doctor about 9 and he came to the house at 11:15. We both thought it was flu, but couldn't be sure.

I couldn't take anything for the diarrhea because if it were chemo-

induced, I needed to get the poisons out. I couldn't take anything for the terrible headache and achiness because we didn't want to mask a fever. If my temperature reached 38 C (100 F), I would have to go to the hospital for blood tests, antibiotics, and an IV. That takes on an added meaning here since it means a Belgian hospital and the need to explain everything in French. I always think of what I want to say after I need to say it, and when I'm feeling bad, my vocabulary disappears.

During the day, several people checked in on me and I drank gallons of Gatorade and tonic when I could hold it down. Bob got home at 4:00—what a relief. I could hardly raise my head off the pillow. By 7:00, my temperature was at 37.6 and I was determined it would not hit 38. By 9:00, I was able to eat some soup, and I slept well last night. This morning, my temperature is normal and I've had a shower and feel pretty good. Thank God it was a twenty-four-hour flu and it was on day nine, before my blood counts are expected to hit their lowest. I'm sure this is far more detail than you ever wanted to know, but it's cathartic to write it.

Once more, I realize how blessed I am that Bob is going through this ordeal with me. To my mother-in-law, Ethel, you should be very proud of the son you raised. He is with me every inch of the way and I feel like "we" have the cancer and the chemo. Thank God he's not like some of the men we all know who leave their families when the going gets rough. I know I couldn't do this without him.

Even the puppy, Sans Souci, was precious yesterday. When I became sick at 4:15, she started crying. Since she is downstairs in the kitchen with the door closed, she usually sleeps through everything. Somehow she sensed things were not right, and she cried until 5:00 when Bob went down to let her out. When he left at 6:30, he put her back in her kennel and I never heard another peep out of her until afternoon when my friend Nancy came and let her out. For the rest of the afternoon, she was in the family room and was an angel. However, when I came downstairs for soup, she decided all was right with the world and she became her usual playful pest-self.

Well, I'm glad it's a new day and I'm ten pounds lighter. Only wish the weight would stay off.

Love,
Barbara

It seemed to me that Chris Georgantopoulos was much more concerned about me than the oncologist. Dr. Kenton did not require any blood work between the chemo treatments. He simply said that if I got sick, I could come to the hospital. In her book, Susan Love wrote that blood tests should be taken about once a week during chemotherapy. If white counts and platelets became too low, GCSF (granulocyte cell stimulating factor) injections would stimulate the recovery of white cells in the bone marrow, thus reducing the threat of infection or risk of bleeding from low platelet counts. While Chris couldn't administer the GCSF, he could monitor the blood counts.

On the Monday following my twenty-four-hour siege, I had a blood test. My white counts were less than half of the pre-chemo level and my absolute neutrophil count was at 640, down from 2620 the week before. Chris said that anything under 1000 was dangerous, and if it hit 500, I would have to hospitalized. He wanted me to have blood drawn every other day, but felt it unsafe for me to come to the military clinic, which was under investigation for a particularly virulent form of staph infection. Therefore, he asked me to wear surgical masks and not stay for physical therapy.

Because my veins were so uncooperative, getting blood was never easy. This was complicated by the fact that I had only one arm to offer. After having the lymph nodes removed, I had to be very careful with my right arm to avoid lymphedema. I could not have injections, blood draws, or blood pressure cuffs on the right arm. In fact, I had been told not to wear a watch on that arm, not to have elastic cuffs, and not to carry a purse on that shoulder. The lab technicians hated to see me coming. On this day, I had two male medics who couldn't find a vein; they handed me off to a female Belgian civilian who finally found one. I felt like a pin cushion.

My family wanted details about the blood counts and I explained as best I understood it myself.

OK—your medical lesson for the day as I understand it—not sure I'd get an A in med school.

The absolute neutrophil is the percentage of white blood cells that actually fight infection. Normal is 40 percent to 74 percent for an absolute count of 1900 - 8000. The day of my first chemo treatment (before I had chemo) my percentage was 49 percent and absolute count was 2620. That's on the low side of normal, but probably indicative of recent surgery, etc. The chemo kills cells— both healthy and cancerous. So at the low point, one must do blood tests to see what the counts look like.

On Monday, my absolute count was 650. If it goes to 500, I have to be hospitalized. I just came back from a blood test this morning, and I'm waiting to get the results by phone. I had to wear a mask in the clinic. If the counts are going back up, I can go to physical therapy. If they are at the same level, I can go if I change masks every ten minutes. If they're down, I can't go anywhere— especially the clinic because it is full of sick people.

Another task that was proving to be anything but easy was the wig. I decided I hated the blonde bowl of curls. Marie called the wig store for me and they said they would exchange it, but not allow it to be returned for credit. I dreaded even going to the shop again since I had been so claustrophobic and stressed there the first time. I ordered several wigs from a catalogue. They would ship them and allow returns. I knew I would be much more comfortable about trying them on in the privacy of my own home. But catalogue ordering from overseas is not always a simple process. The wigs were sent to my office in Virginia and then forwarded to me at the Army Post Office (APO). I worried that they would not arrive before I lost my hair.

Losing my hair caused a lot of stress. I dreamt one night that I went to the wig store to exchange the wig and could not find anything I liked, so I exchanged it for a tablecloth. Bob suggested I could always use the tablecloth like an Arab headdress.

I was having extraordinary dreams. Some were violent, some were upsetting, and all left me shaking and exhausted. One night I had a vivid dream about rain and flood waters that raced through the house. Our belongings washed out into the rain through a front door that looked like the door and vestibule in my childhood home in Maryland. An old man stood and watched, not helping me as I frantically tried to save my things, but offering to build a new vestibule. I wrote to Kennon about the dream, wondering if the rush of water symbolized the chemo. She responded:

February 25, 1997

First I was really fascinated by the connection you made with chemo, which I agree with, so let's assume that the center of your psyche (or God) is trying to tell your ego something about the state of your psyche with chemo. (That's what dreams are, they are "letters" from "God" to the ego about the unconscious part of our life, so that the ego can incorporate the information and use it to affect what is happening in everyday life.)

Your ego's position is "you" in the dream and perhaps we can say the ego is unconsciously very upset, angry, and wants to save those things of value that are threatened. "Those things of value" are the crystal, the furniture, everything heading out the door—but really it is what is represented by these symbols. In other words, don't take literally crystal, furniture, etc., but instead think of all the things you associate with the crystal, each piece of furniture and you'll begin to get a sense of what all is of value and being threatened by the chemo. For instance, maybe the furniture was bought by you and Bob when you were first married, the crystal is a gift from someone—they symbolize feelings or moments of life that could get lost with this illness.

Also, the vestibule and the doors are like Mother's. What do you associate with those? Working with the images in this way, you'll begin to get a sense of what is important and could get damaged by the rain. And by the way, what is "the rain"? Is it a big storm coming, a downpour, a gentle spring rain? Typically rain is a cleansing, but again you have to work with what it is in this dream for you. Can rain cleanse furniture or just damage it?

Also, there is a compensatory aspect to the dream. In real life you have been upbeat and positive—a one-sided attitude toward cancer and the chemo. In the dream you are angry, yelling, very upset—the compensation so that psyche is balanced. In other words, in real life you need to be both positive and angry.

Now, what about the old-fashioned man? He is a hindrance to the efforts of the ego. The ego wants to get all that is valuable back into the house before the rain damages those things. The man does not help and says he will build you a new vestibule. But the vestibule is inside already. What in the world is he talking about? Who is he? He is an aspect of you because he is in your dream. Is he an attitude toward life that has to go—an old-fashioned attitude? If so, what is the attitude? Or is he a part of you that the ego misunderstands and you could elicit to help if done in the right way?

Something called active imagination could be helpful here. Sit down with a pen and paper when you are alone and have a dialogue with him. Ask him questions you want answers to like: Who are you and what are you doing? Why do you want to build me a new vestibule? Why are you not helping me? Write the question and the answer that pops into your mind after you have asked it.

There is a possibility that the chemo is causing a big psychological change in you represented by the furniture flying out the door. The ego is "beside itself" by this, really scared and angry. The old-fashioned man could be helping the psychological change or hindering it. The rain on the contents of the house could be good or bad. The ego has one position about this but not necessarily the correct position. Thus the more you understand the images of the dream, the more you can be open to the psychological changes taking place within, and the ego can "settle down."

By February 28, my blood counts were going down again after one day of going up. Chris was not convinced that the military clinic knew what they were doing in the lab. They did not usually treat oncology patients, but since Dr. Kenton didn't care about my counts, Chris insisted on tracking my blood counts for fear I would get an infection and not be able to fight it off. He thought I would do better going to the local Belgian hospital for blood work. I was at 506 neutrophil count, and Chris was nearly panicked. Ashley was going to the Netherlands on Saturday for the European cheerleading championships, and Bob and I hoped to go watch her. Chris decided that he would go with me Saturday morning to the local Belgian Ambroise Pare Hospital in Mons for blood work. He would get an immediate reading and decide on the spot whether I was to be admitted or could go to see Ashley cheer. Quite a range of choices—and the Netherlands won.

On March 2, I wrote to my e-mail support group:

The oncology nurse predicted I would begin losing my hair on day fifteen and it would all go rapidly. Imagine my delight when day fifteen passed uneventfully. On day sixteen, I saw two hairs on the pillow. On day seventeen, about twelve hairs came out in my comb. Same thing this morning, and since I'm about to go wash my hair, I'm sure that will eliminate a lot. I think I'm ready. I now have four wigs. The ugly blonde bowl of curls will go back to the store this week. The other three are considerably less expensive and look much more natural. After I have to wear them, I'll choose one and send the others back. I've ordered several hats/turbans. And I've practiced with the Hermés scarves. I feel totally inept, but maybe it will come with practice.

The first chemo cycle is almost up. I'll have the second treatment on March 6. I have tolerated it quite well—no chemo-induced nausea at all. I've had continuous fatigue, and I'm glad I'm not working. My blood cell counts went so low that I have been isolated for the last week. I had to wear a surgical mask to go to the clinic for physical therapy and blood work, and otherwise I've stayed home.

It is an interesting sensation to be behind the mask, wondering if people recognize you and knowing they can't see the expression on your face. Some people stare as if you can't see them back. Others avoid looking at you as if you're an alien. One nurse was actually annoyed at me for wearing a mask and demanded to know why. When I told her, she lightened up.

I finally got out of my little world yesterday. After an early morning blood test, Bob and I drove to the Netherlands to see Ashley compete in the all-European cheerleading competition. I was not allowed to go into the gym except for her performance. So, I sat in the car for all but twenty-five minutes out of five hours. But it was worth it. Bob came to get me when Ashley's squad performed, and I stood in the back of the gym with my mask on. Then, I went in again for the awards ceremony to see our school take fifth place in Europe. They were so thrilled. Ashley couldn't see my smile, but she could see the tears in my eyes. Cheerleaders today are athletes, more than just the spirit leaders they were in my day. Ashley is the one who "flies" so she is on the top of the pyramids and is the one thrown high in the air during their stunts. She did a great job.

Thanks for your continuing messages and prayers. Some of you are also sending me funny stories, which I love. I'm sending them on to my brother-in-law who is receiving chemo for colon cancer. So, keep the messages and funny stories coming and the prayers wending their way upwards. Please add Howard to your prayer list as well.

My goddaughter's response was the first suggestion of many, inspiring me to write about my cancer journey.

Your last letter made me cry and laugh, which I'm sure you've been doing a lot of these days. Keeping up your sense of humor is healthy, but letting yourself cry is also.

I was thinking something. You should keep all of these letters and the ones you write and publish them. It really is a phenomenal thing going on. An e-mail diary on your fight against cancer. I'm very serious about this. I think it would be most helpful for a lot of people and it would be a great story to share with millions of people. In any case, I hope you're keeping the letters.

Knowing that humor helps healing and raised my spirits, I started a funny story cancer group. I received jokes from friends Andy and Marjorie, and I began to send them on to Howard and Christine. Christine then sent them on to another friend with cancer. During the months that followed, my funny story cancer group grew. And funny stories came from lots of sources.

However, along with the love, support, humor, and positive attitude, there was still plenty of time for reflection, feelings of despair, and even tears. As the second treatment and hair loss loomed, it helped to know that my supporters understood that too. My cousin Jim put a lot in perspective with another message entitled "Love across the miles."

March 1, 1997

This letter has been in my mind for days as I have remembered you each day in prayer.

I was touched, amused, moved by your "shorn" message. It took me back to the time when Judy got the word that she would be getting chemotherapy. She went out and bought a wig, just in case. When she brought it home and tried it on, she looked like a little girl playing dress-up. As it turned out she didn't lose but a tiny amount of hair and the wig remained in the closet. It sounds like you are taking a more aggressive treatment and that you will probably lose the hair.

For me the whole matter of losing a breast and losing hair was all tied up with how we face loss, period. A person relates to his/her lover and friend in a very bodily way and so the loss of any portion of that person's body is bound to cause some trauma and some sadness. I remember when Judy took the bandages off and was in the bathtub. She called me in and I saw her as I had not seen her before. The surprise for me was that I did not fall apart; in fact, I could see nothing but this strong, beautiful, very wonderful woman in front of me. I had seen a whole collection of pictures of women without one or both breasts and, at the time, I had even felt a special beauty in them. Seeing Judy confirmed the feeling for myself.

As far as the hair is concerned, there is a whole different approach that believes in going bald. The late André Lorde, writer and poet, wrote some marvelous stuff about the challenge and dignity of going public, even defying convention. It's not for everyone, but it touched me when I read it while Judy was fearing losing that part of her body she prizes the most—her hair.

Jim, himself an author and preacher of huge talent, had put great assurance into beautiful words. I mean, how sexy can a woman be with one breast, a huge scar, wearing over-sized t-shirts or pajama tops, and going bald? I figured I needed to take the bull by the horns. I had read about a woman who had dressed and undressed in the closet for many years after her mastectomy, never allowing her husband to see or touch her. That wasn't for me, but the longer I waited to have "show and tell," the more difficult it became.

One night, I simply said to Bob, "You need to look at me without clothes on."

He agreed and I removed my pajama top. He leaned over and kissed the ugly scar, and that was that. Nothing's easy, but that was easier than I expected.

83

The Fourth Chakra

Ethel Soriano is a holistic healer and friend of my sister, Kennon. They do research together and occasionally practice and present workshops on dream analysis in Mexico City where Ethel lives and practices. Ethel has studied with native healers in Central and South America. When Ethel learned that both Howard and I had cancer, she prepared several things to help us through the treatment. First, she sent Bach Flower Remedy based on my particular "transit chart." By knowing the time and date of my birth, and utilizing the work of Dr. Edward Bach coupled with Jung's archetypes, Ethel was able to prescribe very specific flower essences that are most effective in a certain moment of time in a person's life. For me, the essences of gentian, honeysuckle, holly, elm, and chicory were applicable during the first chemo cycle.

Ethel also sent a balance chakra sensor, a wire of seven stones representing the seven chakras of the body. The semiprecious stones were red, orange, yellow, green, blue, indigo, and violet, representing the full range of colors of the rainbow that are visible to the naked eye. Ethel explained that one uses the wire like worry beads, turning the stones in both directions to direct energy into the particular chakras or to remove blockages in areas of the body. Chakra four pertained to my problems. I was amazed when I saw the description for chakra four.

Organs: heart and circulatory system; lungs; shoulders and arms; ribs and breasts; diaphragm; thymus gland.

Mental and emotional issues: love and hatred; resentment and bitterness; grief; self-centeredness; loneliness and commitment; forgiveness and compassion; hope and trust.

Physical dysfunctions: congestive heart failure; myocardial infarction (heart attack); mitral valve prolapse; cardiomegaly; asthma/allergy; lung cancer; bronchial pneumonia; upper back; shoulder; breast cancer.

The similarity of that description for chakra four compared to my health history was incredible. Nine years earlier, I had been diagnosed with mitral valve prolapse. For the past nine years, I had taken an antibiotic when I visited the dentist to prevent contaminated blood from backtracking through the mitral valve and into my heart. Interestingly, the MUGA scan showed no mitral valve prolapse, so it may have been a misdiagnosis. Currently, I had tendinitis in my shoulder on the mastectomy side, and I was being treated for breast cancer.

Considering the emotional issues, I was certainly lonely. The treatment caused me to be very self-centered. I needed to trust my doctors and have hope for the best. The heart was indicated on both organs and physical dysfunctions. I had experienced high blood pressure several times during my life. It was the high blood pressure that had fortuitously led me to Chris Georgantopoulos.

The fourth stone was a beautiful green malachite. I had always loved malachite and I had several pieces of malachite jewelry. In fact, my friend and mentor, Max, who had died of leukemia, had given me malachite earrings from South America. This all seemed like an omen.

Along with this package of holistic remedies, Kennon sent a beautiful silver pin of a shaman, herbs to strengthen the immune system during chemo, and several more books to read. As I was preparing for the second session of chemo, I decided that my symbols should go with me for the treatment, even as I had the table of symbols when I was hospitalized. Because the most active poison in the chemo was red, I made a point of wearing red every time I received chemo. Into my jacket pocket, I put the cross that read "*Je suis avec vous*" and the wire of stones representing the chakras, and I wore the shaman pin.

On our way to the *hopital du jour*, Bob and I stopped at the wig shop to exchange the bowl of blonde curls. As I tried on various wigs, I noticed that more and more hair came out on my blazer. I was shedding unbelievably. That made me incredibly anxious as I tried on wigs. I looked at a red one, thinking that perhaps redheaded Ashley and I could pretend to be twins. I finally opted for a light-brown, short wig without much curl, but I didn't like it very well either. Since I couldn't get a refund, and they didn't have table cloths as in my dream, I just had to get anything. As we left the shop and walked down the street, Bob reached over and touched the back of my head. His hand came away holding a huge clump of hair. I wondered if I would make it through the chemo treatment with any hair on my head.

At Jules Bordet, we had the required blood draw after three attempts to find a vein, and then went to see Dr. Kenton. He was perfunctory in asking the required questions about health during the previous three weeks. He seemed unconcerned that I had been sick and thought Chris was overreacting to make me wear a mask. He didn't care what my blood counts had been. This day's blood test showed that my cell counts had not completely regenerated, but Dr. Kenton said to go ahead and receive chemo anyway since we had driven from Mons.

He also gave me an anti-inflammatory medication for the tendinitis in my shoulder. Despite the physical therapy, my shoulder was getting worse instead of better, constantly painful, even sore to the touch. I could not sleep on that side, and I was losing range of motion. In fact, it hurt so much that I often lost sleep. I wondered if the physical therapy might be causing the problems, but Marie thought I was not mobile enough, so she was stretching the living daylights out of me.

We talked about whether it might be possible for me to travel to Williamsburg during the third week of this cycle. I had Alumni Board meetings at William and Mary, and I had not missed a full board meeting in five years. I really wanted to go. Dr. Ward had told me I should not fly during the AC chemo regimen, but Dr. Kenton said if I felt all right and did not run a fever during this cycle, I could go after day fifteen. He gave me a prescription for antibiotics to start taking the day before I left and cautioned that if I ran a fever, I should go immediately to the hospital. Then he sent me off for round two.

Patients receiving chemotherapy in the *hopital du jour* were each given a private room. I would sit on the bed and Bob would sit in a chair. The oncology nurse would start the IV drips and would come and go except when the Adriamycin was being administered. Because it was so toxic, the nurse would put on rubber gloves and administer the entire bag, very carefully checking the flow to be sure it was going into the veins and not backing up. The whole process took about an hour. Bob and I would read, or I would close my eyes and rest. We didn't feel much like talking. I always felt a certain detachment as I watched the deadly chemicals dripping into my veins.

I didn't know whether my symbols were helping me any, but it made the chemotherapy into a ritual. For me, rituals and traditions help to define significant events. I remembered that when Max was having his deadliest chemo and had set up his table of symbols, he asked Ashley to draw him a purple amoeba. He posted it on his wall and said he would look at it and remember that the purple amoeba, representing the chemicals, was his friend. By pushing him closer to death through killing both the cancer and the good cells in his body, it also gave him a chance for life. The symbols in my pockets served that purpose for me.

Mistakenly, I concentrated my attention on the fourth stone of the balance chakra sensor that Ethel had sent me, the green malachite. When I reported that to Ethel, she wrote to correct my error. She explained that the fourth chakra had too much energy or an energy blockage, and that I should work with blue, not green, in order to balance the energy throughout my body. According to chromotherapy, blue would control the activity of the cells to stop malignant growth; it would also decrease pain. Ethel suggested that I wear blue jewelry, not the green malachite. She also suggested that I cover a lamp with blue cellophane and let the blue light shine on the surgical area and the affected shoulder. In another package, Ethel sent a bag of raw aquamarine for me to carry with me.

The chemo had a cumulative effect. I did not experience the terrible nausea that many chemo patients suffer, and the anti-nausea medication was a godsend. But, I felt the increasing fatigue. On most days, I did little more than go to physical therapy and come home and take a nap. I had made the decision that I would not try to work. After the required three months, I applied for disability insurance payments. The insurance would pay my salary, and VIMA would receive a credit for the insurance premium for my policy. That proved to be a good move. It took a lot of pressure off me so that I could just concentrate on healing. And it relieved the company of the financial burden of supporting me for six of the nine months that I was not working.

I continued to communicate with VIMA daily by e-mail, but they knew to take actions without waiting for my guidance. My e-mail support group included all my VIMA colleagues, and they could be more productive if they knew that I was getting through the treatment and preparing to come back to the company at a later time. After the second round of chemo, I wrote to my support group:

March 7

Some of you have wondered if it is okay to tell others about my cancer—absolutely yes. All this feeling of love from others helps me stay positive about the treatment.

On Wednesday night, I attended my first meeting of the breast cancer support group here. There are about eight ladies, mostly British and American, one Turk, and an Italian lady whom I took with me who had just been diagnosed. It was wonderful to talk to these ladies who are at various stages of treatment between new diagnosis and just reaching their five-year anniversary without recurrence— a major landmark. We shared stories, catalogues of post-surgical products, experiences with different treatments, and it was great to feel not alone in the experience. Also an interesting bond across nationalities. We all have the same fears, pains, and hopes when it comes to the breast cancer.

I had my second chemo session yesterday. I've decided to wear red every day I get chemo—a red blazer on the first time and a red blouse yesterday. Red is the symbolic color of Saint Barbara, patron saint of the artillery, engineers, fire fighters and those who deal with explosives. So, I imagine that Saint Barbara is directing these fighters, surging through my body and firing on the enemy. How's that for symbolism? I tolerated the chemo well, the anti-nausea medication is working and I feel fine today. It is also six weeks after the surgery, and most of the two doses of general anesthesia are out of my body, so I'm feeling better in that regard.

In the last message, I told you that my hair was "Going, going..." Now it's gone. After yesterday's chemo, the hair said, "Enough is enough." Just touching my hair caused huge clumps to come out in my hand. So, last night, I gently pulled as much out as I could. This morning, I cut what was left very close to the scalp. It is simply a mess to have hair all over the place. So, today is day one with the wig. When I went to the hospital for physical therapy, I got lots of compliments about my new hair do. When I explained it wasn't mine, most people expressed surprise. Either they were being polite, or this wig is pretty good. We were able to exchange the awful blonde curls I had bought previously for something more natural and easier to care for. Ashley thinks I should get a green punk wig—right.

It was incredible to stand in front of the mirror and pull my hair out. It didn't hurt at all. It just came out in huge handfuls. For days, it had been clogging the shower drains. It was all over the towels. Even though I wore a sleep cap at night, it was all over the pillow. When I did laundry, it got all over the clothes. Maybe I should have shaved my head. Even with it as short as I had it cut, it was simply a mess. By pulling it out, I could avoid some of the mess. Eventually, I decided to shave off the remainder. Thank heavens it was finally gone. The anticipation of losing my hair turned out to be worse than actually losing it. I never had the nerve to go bald, and neither Bob nor Ashley ever saw me without something on my head. When I did not wear the wig, the red turban became my favorite head covering. I slept in it and wore it around the house when no one else was there. But, when I looked in the mirror I confronted my own bald head without terrible feelings. As Kennon had said, I couldn't hide. My essence stared right back at me.

Losing one's hair is a rite of passage in cancer treatment. It raises questions of what is important in life. It is symbolic of letting go. It is almost an act of cleansing, in preparation for new growth. Kennon's next gift to me symbolized this search. Along with two wonderful and colorful Mexican dolls, she wrote:

One night in Puebla, Ethel and I went to an organ concert in a church near where we were staying. I don't particularly like organ music because it is so solemn, and all during the concert, I thought about you and Howard. I started crying quietly and felt so discouraged about life. The concert was performed by a young music student and that made me think about youth and the potential within us that we are all so aware of as students and in young adulthood. I thought about how that potential changes and I pondered the question, how do we understand and let the passage of time take us to other stages of our life without trying to hold on to earlier times?

When we left, I was feeling rather low, and as we walked I saw this family sitting on a blanket under a tree. It was 10 o'clock at night, the children were asleep, as was the father, and there sat the mother and grandmother making dolls with colorful ribbons all across their heads. I was filled with the sensation of how these dolls were such a celebration of life.

The mother and grandmother had such a simple life—this was where they were sleeping for the next few days until they sold their dolls and could go back to their village—and yet their faces were bright with smiles and happiness. I could not resist buying you these two dolls, and now I'm sending them to you with all the spirit of a celebration of life that I felt that night. It was like a gift to me from these women and now I am sending it to you.

Celebrating life became a challenge during the downward spiral of chemotherapy. With each passing day, more mysteries confronted me, but I determined I would get through this and on to what might become a deeper and happier place.

Keeping Up With the Glacels

Arriving home from the second round of chemo at Jules Bordet, an e-mail message from friends Lynne and Andy entitled "Keeping up with the Glacels" greeted us. Andy had been regularly sending me funny stories and keeping me laughing. We had known Lynne and Andy since 1981 when Bob and Andy were majors together at the Army Command and General Staff College in Kansas. From there, both families had moved to Alaska and lived just two blocks apart. Their daughters had baby-sat for our girls, and both families had camped together often.

After Alaska, we all moved to Virginia and lived within five miles of each other. In fact, when Lynne and Andy arrived a year after we had moved to Virginia, they lived in our club basement for some weeks waiting to move into their home. We had shared season tickets at the Kennedy Center for years. What could they mean by "keeping up" with us?

As I read, I became shocked and distressed. Andy wrote:

March 5, 1997

Subject: Keeping up with the Glacels
I can't be totally outdone by you.
I will say your being open and communicative about your cancer is and has been inspirational.
So much so that I had to go out and get one myself.
We (Lynne and I) just got back from the Dr. and I was told that I have cancer of the prostate. Since I didn't even know what it was (or that I had one) it took a while to explain. It was noted by the annual PSA test (slightly high) and "bend over" (slightly enlarged—

—that worried me because nothing there has ever been large). Subsequent sonogram showed nothing, biopsy showed positive signs.

Will be getting bone scan to determine spread and then will schedule surgery.

I am pretty positive about what I know and what needs to be done.

Honestly, your openness has been a MAJOR help in my understanding and acceptance.

Will keep you posted.

Andy

I was stunned. In fact, I had to read the message twice because I didn't get it when Andy said, "I had to go out and get one myself." I responded immediately, with tears in my eyes:

Andy,

That is not the way to keep up with anyone. But if I have to share experiences, I'm glad it is with a friend—only wish it were positive experiences. Actually, there is some positive to everything. Friends and support come out of the woodwork. I'll put you on my funny story list, but I think lots of them have originated with you. I'm collecting more, though. Please, please keep us informed of what you learn and your treatment. You're in our prayers. We've learned that cancer is a family illness, so we pray, too, for Lynne, Shawn, Kim and Christy.

I did not know whether there were more people being diagnosed with cancer these days or whether I was simply more attuned to it because it consumed my life at the moment. It seemed to be an epidemic. Somehow, I felt more anger at Andy's diagnosis of cancer than I had felt about my own. Lynne wrote:

March 11, 1997

The big 'C.':

You provided a great example for Andy. When we were told of the diagnosis, one of Andy's first questions was "OK, who/how do we tell?" The who, of course, family and close friends, but having witnessed the strength you gained from being open and forthright with everyone left no question in either of our minds that Andy should follow your example. So far it seems to help a lot. Knowing everyone cares is wonderful. Andy is receiving calls not only from our friends, but friends of friends. I am amazed at the number of men walking around without prostates—an organ I knew nothing about two weeks ago.

Andy is an 'okay, lets get this done' kind of guy. This learn, test, wait, learn, test…is hard, but I think he is doing well.

Andy's diagnosis made me realize how my own support group felt being so far away from me. I lived nearly 4000 miles away from Andy. What could I do? I shifted my funny story group into high gear. I had been sending occasional jokes and stories, but I decided that now I would send one every day. Howard was having a very hard time with his chemo and needed to laugh. Andy needed to laugh his way through this time of uncertainty, as did Christine, waiting for a new experimental chemo to arrive from the States. So, I made us official.

March 9

To Howard, Andy, Christine,

You all know from my last message that I have dubbed us the "funny story cancer group." That's how your addresses are listed in my e-mail address book. But, I'm the only common link, so you must meet each other.

Howard, my brother-in-law of about twenty-six years, lives in Chicago and has colon cancer. Howard starts his third round of chemo on Monday, March 10. When his counts are good, he goes to Oregon where he works on architectural projects.

Andy, my Army friend of about fifteen years, lives in Fairfax, Virginia. Our families have lived together in Kansas, Alaska, and Virginia. We have shared children, cars, camping, and season tickets at the Kennedy Center. Andy was just diagnosed with prostate cancer. Andy is the originator of the funny stories being sent to me, and I hope I don't send any back to you, Andy.

Christine is my new friend in Brussels. Christine is an American, married to a diplomat from the Netherlands, and has lived all around Europe. Christine had breast cancer twelve years ago and is now receiving chemo for a tumor on her liver. Christine helped me with wig shopping and has good advice. She is also sharing the stories with another friend who has ovarian cancer.

I was reminded yesterday by Christine's and my mutual friend, Mieke, about Norman Cousins who "laughed himself well by watching old Marx Brothers movies." Let's follow his lead—at least one good belly laugh a day. Okay?

The funny story for today should ring a bell for all of us travelers.

I had enlisted the aid of my e-mail support group to send jokes and funny stories, and they were coming in great numbers. There were down days for each of us when the only laughs for the funny story group came from our e-mail stories. Howard wrote with more enthusiasm than I had heard from him in a long time, "Keep them coming." Christine wrote, "Laughed myself sick with the story on the soap bars."

Somehow the combination of the e-mail discussion about losing my hair and the request for funny stories persuaded some in my support group to send funny hats. Sarah sent a bushy, fake-fur hat from St. Petersburg that tied under my chin. Ashley brought me a straw summer hat from an Easter trip to the Ukraine. Anne sent a sequined red, white, and blue baseball cap. But the funniest hat came from Jim in Bermuda. He wrote:

I am glad you emphasized that laughter is the best medicine. I picked up something for you in town here (a bit of local color), then was afraid you might be put off by the silliness of it. I will get it in the mail to you the first of the week.

When the mail arrived, to my delight, Jim had sent a knit hat with rastafarian-style dreadlocks. It surely met my need for hair, and I got a wonderful chuckle at the "Rasta Imposta."

I also learned that breast cancer patients can find great healing by laughing at ourselves. I had been attending the international breast cancer support group with a Turkish woman who had just finished chemotherapy. Before she started radiation, she went to Turkey to see her family who did not know of her diagnosis and treatment. Greeted by her family with great excitement, she prepared for a large family dinner in her honor. Her uncle picked her up and, unable to find a parking place, he impatiently honked the horn. Sukran, who had just gotten out of the shower, quickly threw on her clothes. After she arrived to the restaurant and greeted the extended family, she looked down at herself and loudly exclaimed, "Oh my God, I forgot my breast!" Sure enough, she had left the prosthesis back in her bedroom, and she appeared very lopsided. That softened the blow of the news to her family, and an aunt took her to the ladies' room where they stuffed her bra full of toilet paper.

With that story, Sukran had us all in hysterics. It was so healthy. Only cancer patients can find humor in our situation. Others would never dream of laughing at cancer. But, as with all aspects of life, there is humor even in cancer.

Kennon had mentioned to me that I needed to deal with anger as well as with humor. In her earlier dream analysis, she thought that my anger was coming out in my dreams. I wrote to her:

> *I finished reading* Cancer as Initiation *last night. The last chapters were good and quite interesting. As the author told about healing, it wasn't so heavy and I could read it more consistently. There was one footnote that started me thinking. She talked about the negative role of hostility in healing. I realized that there have been several things that have happened where I could have felt real anger, but haven't:*
>
> - *The doctor in Germany who told me not to have a mammogram last November. I think he's an idiot, but I'm not angry with him.*
> - *I've not experienced the "Why me?" anger at God or my body.*
> - *When I was sent home from the hospital instead of having surgery on the original day scheduled—I actually enjoyed the weekend at home.*
> - *When more cancer was found and I had to have a second operation. I think the doctor was more distraught than I was.*
>
> *The closest I came to anger was at the woman oncologist who wouldn't talk to us. But, I'm okay with the man I'm seeing and I haven't held on to that anger. I think all of that has helped me.*
>
> *Another insight I had was about dreams. Barbara Stone talks about dreaming of pregnancy, revealing the birth of the "new" her.*

I actually had dreams for some time before diagnosis about being caught out in public bare-breasted. Maybe it is too literal to say that was a message about breast cancer, but I wonder?

Kennon responded:

Your insight about anger made me think about your dream that we have not followed up on. Remember that I said your anger in the dream was a compensation for the outer attitude of being so positive. If we are one-sided in an attitude, the psyche has to balance the one-sidedness in the unconscious which is where dreams come from. When I read the list of things that have made you angry but then you had a reason in each circumstance to not be angry, it made me think about our family. We never learned how to be angry. Instead I think you and I adopted Mother's attitude which is to find the good in something.

Anger is a very important emotion. When felt properly and utilized it gives one strength, direction, and health. Only in the last few years have I learned how to express anger in a relationship (not in an out-of-control way) and learned that without the expression of it, the relationship becomes neutral. If you can try to forget the positive twist you put on things for a moment and just let yourself be angry, knowing that the other person will not collapse or be offended for life, you will feel anger.

For instance, the doctor who told you not to have a mammogram—and who also did not hear that your father had high blood pressure and died from it: yes he is stupid but also can you make a clear, angry statement that his inattention to life-threatening problems in your body makes you angry? You don't have to call him up and scream at him, you just have to feel within yourself red-hot anger and hold it consciously. Tell yourself or Bob how angry his inattention to detail made you because you could have died from it. Be angry at him. Much later you can resolve within yourself that he is a dope or overworked or had a bad day or whatever you want to rationalize but not until you have been angry at him. This applies to each of the incidents you cited. And go back to your dream to see how angry you were. That gives you the realization of how angry you really are. Anger is not a bad thing.

I am impressed with the things you are thinking about. Your thoughts about the dreams of being bare-breasted are right-on. In such a dream you would want to ask what is being revealed, and to answer the question we always have to include the physical body. Howard had a dream in October that in retrospect told what was happening to him. The dream was that he is in the top of a very tall cedar tree just off the deck of the house he was renovating on Canterbury Street in Portland. He was in the tree, cutting out branches so that there was a better view of Mt. Hood from the deck of the house (which is like a tree house). Suddenly he realized that at the bottom of the cedar tree someone with a saw was cutting down the tree and that he would topple over with it. A tree is a very strong symbol of the self. Marie Louise von Franz, a Jungian analyst in Zurich, wrote a book called Dreams and Death *in which she examines dreams that lead us to ask about our bodily health.*

Well, BP, you are doing great and if you can get angry you will be doing even better. Ethel is so impressed with how you are working with the cancer and she wanted me to tell you.

The second round of chemo was uneventful in terms of any illness. I continued to do more driving, and as clothes became more comfortable, I even did some of my own shopping. Friends had been helpful about picking up things at the store for me, so I hadn't had to make the thirty-mile drive to the American shopping facilities. I knew, though, that if I was serious about going to Williamsburg during the third week of this cycle that I should try to do more things and see how I felt. Chris continued to track my blood counts, but was a little more relaxed as he saw that I was not getting sick.

After physical therapy one day, I decided to drive to the American facilities. I retrieved dry cleaning, picked up my airline ticket for the trip to Williamsburg, and then went to the grocery store where I walked blindly into a closed glass door. I was not hurt, but embarrassed. And I had an absolute fight or flight stress reaction—wanting only to flee home and to bed. This experience was my first realization of the chemo fog surrounding me and dimming my awareness. I felt very fragile.

I actually experienced a lot of anxiety about going to Williamsburg, but I wanted to go. I had been on the Board of Directors of the College of

William and Mary Society of the Alumni for five years. Despite living in California, Virginia, and then Belgium, I had never missed a meeting until the January executive committee meeting. This would be my last year on the board.

In preparation for the trip, I planned for many logistical details that would not otherwise concern me. The executive secretary helped me far beyond the call of duty, to include finding names of local doctors whom I could call in case of emergency. She also told me that she thought most board members did not know I was being treated for cancer. That surprised me, since the cancer was the reason I had missed the executive committee meeting in January. But, I suppose it is hard to give bad news and perhaps even harder for men to talk about a female colleague's breast. I cared about the people on the board and had worked with them for five years. I needed their understanding and support if I were to travel to Williamsburg for the meeting in the middle of my treatment.

I asked the executive secretary to tell as many people as possible before my arrival, which would make confronting people I hadn't seen for a while an easier task. After all, if they were to learn the news publicly, it would be embarrassing for them and awkward for me. What exactly does one say in these circumstances? "Hi, haven't seen you for a while, and I'm bald now." I wouldn't be able to hug and kiss people, and shouldn't even shake hands, so it was easier if people knew in advance.

As I prepared for the trip, the anxiety of travel and the perhaps irrational feeling that I was not important enough to my boardmates for them to be informed of my illness finally evoked some of the anger that Kennon had encouraged me to get out. I wrote to tell Kennon:

March 16, 1997
Last night I cried a lot for the first time in ages. I wonder, is it because I'm feeling anger? Is it because I didn't take a nap yesterday? Is it because my counts are dropping this week? Is it because I'm actually quite stressed about going to the States?

The anger did not feel good and only depressed me. Maybe it wasn't just anger I was feeling. It was real hurt and disappointment. I needed support. I needed people to help me through this hard time. Why would anyone want to "keep up with the Glacels," as Andy had said, when I felt so bad? So, as Kennon had commented, I did what Mother always did and tried to turn it into something positive. I would get to go to Williamsburg, see Jenn, and take her to her favorite restaurant, the Trellis, for a very late birthday lunch. But Kennon responded:

> *I feel so badly for you, but I want to raise some questions again. Many religions and philosophies believe that nothing happens by chance, so if you and I consider the possibility of this thought, it might help with understanding what is going on at this moment in your life.*
>
> *Your crying may have had to do with feeling so awful about yourself. You try so hard, you are so responsible, so thorough, so good in your work, you have lots of achievements—so what's wrong? Are you crying because everything at times seems hopeless? I am not assuming that what I am saying is true, but since we cannot have a dialogue about it that would let you confirm what rings true, I'm just proceeding with these thoughts and you can confirm them or throw them out as you read them.*
>
> *You wondered if you really want to go to Williamsburg now. And you noted that your cell count is going down. Is this a good time for you to travel? Think about your health right now and nothing else. If it gives you life spirit and energy to go to Williamsburg, then go, but if you are going for a reason that is fading, think about not going.*

Did Williamsburg give me life spirit and energy? Yes, definitely, as did seeing my friends and colleagues at VIMA. I would not get to see all the important people in my life, but the trip would be worth it if I didn't get sick. It seemed worth the risk, even at a time when I found myself avoiding risk.

Road Trip

Travel has always been one of my greatest joys, so it was strange to face this trip with great apprehension. I had barely left my house for three months, and here I was making a trans-Atlantic flight in the midst of chemo treatment. Dr. Ward had cautioned that this wasn't a good idea. Dr. Kenton had said it was fine if I weren't running a fever. I had blood work done the day before, and the neutrophil count was around 1100, so Chris gave me the go-ahead.

My friend Linda drove to Dulles Airport to pick me up. She became my guardian angel for the weekend. We stopped in briefly at VIMA for a wonderful, but awkward, reunion. We are accustomed to hugging each other when we have been apart for a while, but I didn't want to touch anyone. They saw me for the first time in my physically altered state and with a wig, but everyone handled it well, even without touching.

Linda and I arrived in Williamsburg in time for me to attend meetings. I tried to be upbeat and direct, but clearly my cancer was a difficult subject to be discussed. I did fine through the two days of meetings, opting out of afternoon tours so I could nap. One night we attended a large dinner of several hundred people. I did not shake hands, creating an awkwardness at greeting others. I passed it off lightly, laughing and saying, "I'm not shaking hands these days." Most people would, of course, then ask why. As I had predicted, the answer caused embarrassment to the other person who did not know how to respond..

Linda and I stayed in Williamsburg for another night, and it did nurture my spirit that craved contact with loved ones. We went to dinner with a dear friend, Carolyn, who had been assistant dean of women when I was a student at William and Mary. She helped Bob and me find a place to live when we married in the middle of my senior year and I had to move off campus.

On Saturday, we had our annual Trellis lunch with Jenn and her sorority sisters. This had become a tradition for Jenn's birthday. Although this celebration was six weeks late, it helped make up for my missing her twenty-first birthday. Joining us was another long-time friend whose husband had waged a courageous fight against lung cancer and had died just as we were moving to Belgium in 1995. Owners of the Trellis, Marcel and Connie Desaulniers, treated us to champagne and a wonderful assortment of Death by Chocolate Trellis desserts after our meal. Good thing I did not have the nausea associated with chemo.

When Linda and I returned to northern Virginia, we had a full schedule before I flew back to Belgium on Monday. Linda had researched buying a prosthesis. I had panicked so about a prosthesis in January, but after Madame Carstairs had rescued me, I had been very happy wearing the soft, cotton prosthesis she had made for me. I had not gone out enough in Belgium to worry about wearing anything, and in Williamsburg, I felt fine with this temporary and comfortable form. Certainly I had not felt enough need for a permanent one to tackle buying a prosthesis in a foreign language.

Linda learned where we could go for a fitting and that I should wear a form-fitting sweater rather than a loose blouse. Both Linda and the fitter were very concerned with my privacy. The fitter brought several different prostheses and mastectomy bras, showed me how to insert the prosthesis, and then left me to get it on myself. My shoulder problems, however, prevented me from reaching behind me. So I would get the bra positioned, tell the fitter it was okay, and she would come back into the dressing room to hook the bra. Then I would put the sweater on and model for Linda. The three of us decided on the right size. I wanted a prosthesis with velcro strips that could actually be attached right to my chest with corresponding adhesive velcro, and they had to order that.

The mastectomy bras were unattractive and very wide between the two cups. I commented on this, but the fitter did not know why. She suggested that I could buy any bras in stock and they would sew pockets into them. I bought two mastectomy bras and two pretty, lacy bras that they would alter and mail with the prosthesis. When those bras actually arrived and I tried to use them, I discovered why there needed to be a wide connection between the two cups. The prosthesis, when not velcroed to one's skin, sits in the bra pocket and is heavy. Therefore, it needs the tight, wide fabric to keep the cup close to one's chest. After buying the lovely lacy bras, I did not wear them very often because it always felt as though the prosthesis was flopping away from my chest. But I learned that later, so at the time I was happy with my purchases.

Before returning to Belgium, I spent a day at Walter Reed with the medical professionals who had come to my rescue by phone back in January. I met Dr. Dave Jaques, the surgeon who called me on the night of my diagnosis; Dr. Lou Diehl, the oncologist who guided me through the chemotherapy decision; and Jane Shotkin, the oncology nurse who prepared me for the side effects of the chemo. I spent a long time with Dr. Diehl and found him to be an incredible, patient, caring physician. During the three months of my treatment, he was always available by phone, even initiating calls to me on occasion just to ask about my progress. He obviously knew and empathized with both the emotional and physical effects of chemotherapy. He drew diagrams for me and wrote down the facts he was telling me, so I did not have to take notes or remember. He explained fully why the Americans wanted me to have both chemotherapy and tamoxifen. Interestingly, he and the Belgians cited the same studies, but the interpretation differed. Very few studies had been done at that time with patients having both treatments, but the small sample showed a 7 percent difference in the rate of recurrence for patients with only chemo, or only tamoxifen, compared to both treatments in succession. The Belgians concluded that with such a low percentage difference, chemo was not necessary. The Americans concluded that a 7 percent difference warranted the stronger treatment. I suppose the jury is out on whether the Adriamycin might be more harmful in the long run, but I also wondered if the difference in interpretation signaled any different value on individual lives. Or even if it symbolized the lack of individual attention under a socialized-medicine, managed-care system. At any rate, I wanted to be on the right side of the 7 percent difference.

Equally welcoming, Dr. Jaques expressed delight that I had healed enough from the surgery to travel. I must admit that I got teary when I met him. He had been my first lifeline when I received the bad news, and he had been so compassionate. In my experience, I have found that some doctors deal so much with serious illness that they take it too lightly. They don't seem to remember that, for the patient, this is a new and shocking diagnosis. Dr. Jaques seemed to remember that each patient had tremendous psychological needs when cancer was diagnosed. When I learned a year later that he was leaving Walter Reed for Memorial Sloan Kettering, I told him that if I ever had a recurrence, I would want him to be my doctor wherever he might be.

Jane Shotkin, in real life, proved to be as helpful as she had been on e-mail. She liked my wig, and she talked about other head coverings. She expressed concern about my shoulder, which was increasingly more painful. She referred me to a physical therapist at the Bethesda Naval Hospital who dealt specifically with breast cancer patients and who would consult with Marie on my treatment.

On the way from Walter Reed to Dulles Airport for my return flight to Belgium, Linda and I stopped to buy a mastectomy bathing suit. Determined to get me away from the site of illness, Bob had planned a trip to Portugal during the next cycle if, again, I could travel. We found only one possible bathing suit, so it would have to do if I went swimming in Portugal.

With great relief, I boarded the plane back to Belgium. The trip had raised my spirits but had tired me out too. I could never have done it without Linda's loving care. Of course I could drive or shop or care for myself, but then the fatigue took over and the chemo fog made me inattentive to detail. Driving on my own would not have been safe. Truly, Linda had been my guardian angel.

On my return to Belgium, I found a large envelope in the mail. VIMA belonged to the Instructional Systems Association, a professional trade association, in which I had been very active as a board member. The annual four-day conference in March allowed the best business education and sharing I had ever experienced, as well as fun with wonderful colleagues and competitors. The dates of the conference coincided with the low point of my chemo cycle, so I missed this meeting.

I knew that my condition and absence were mentioned at the opening session by the conference chair because I immediately received e-mail from several folks who had laptops with them. These were upbeat messages from folks whom I knew once a year through business, but who sent heartfelt messages when they heard I was ill.

The large envelope awaiting me had been mailed from the ISA headquarters, further evidence of the positive energy I could feel coming to me from friends and colleagues. Nine pages of large newsprint had been filled with personal messages, doodled drawings, prayers, concerns, and hopes to see me at the next year's conference. I cried as I read each personal message and knew that my presence had been missed by my colleagues. The conference chair wrote to me:

> It was great fun to do the flipcharts, Barbara. We had them plastered across the back of the room, and you would have loved seeing everyone standing back there during breaks writing messages to you. Hope all is well.

It is interesting now to read those messages and note that three of the women who signed my giant card have been subsequently diagnosed with breast cancer.

The Chemo Fog

Driving to Jules Bordet in Brussels for chemo was always a somber event. As we approached the hospital, I would look up at the windows of the surgical ward and imagine some woman lying there, having just come down from the operating room, in pain, wondering if the surgeon got all the cancer, what her follow-on treatments would be, scared about whether she might die. I found it depressing. Outside the hospital was a huge medieval building called the *Porte de Hal*, the only remaining gate of the second fortification of the town, built between 1357 and 1383. As we approached the *Porte de Hal* on every visit, it somehow felt like stepping back in time.

The dark and dreary buildings of the hospital nestled between other unimaginative and massive structures. The typically overcast Belgian weather joined the surroundings to cast a pall on the entrance. Just as the *Porte de Hal* made me step back in time, I also felt as though time stopped when I entered Bordet. In fact, the cancer diagnosis and treatment made me feel as though I had hit a wall while going at breakneck speed. Life as I knew it had stopped. Cancer put the skids on normal routine. Even the trip to Williamsburg did not break that spell as I went to Bordet for the third round of chemo on the day following my return.

I arrived decked out in a red shirt with a red and black blazer to match the red Adriamycin. Saint Barbara lived vividly in my imagination. After several unsuccessful sticks, the technician drew my blood and we discovered that my counts had not regenerated back to normal. Bob and I were both afraid the treatment would be delayed, but the oncologist said the counts were close enough for me to receive the chemo. He warned, however, that perhaps the next session would have to be delayed. Off we went to the *hopital du jour*, where once again, my veins did not cooperate. Three sticks and two nurses later, I had an IV running. While I received the chemo, Bob read to me about the history and tourism in Normandy, France. If I avoided the nausea as I had for the past two treatments, we would spend Easter weekend at a bed and breakfast in Normandy.

The chemotherapy had a definite cumulative effect. With each treatment, I dropped a little lower because I had not quite rebounded from the last treatment. This treatment seemed even worse because my counts were so low when I received it. My cousin Jim's wife, Judy, wrote:

> *Do you not feel special being under the chemo spell? I used to think what an awesome experience. It will pass quickly. The three months will be over soon.*

It was heartening to hear her message, but it did not feel that way as I lived the experience. However, I never thought that I made the wrong decision. My friend Jean told me an interesting story. Her mother had died of breast cancer almost twenty years before. Her mother and Betty Ford had their cancer surgery in the same hospital on the same day. Their tumors were staged exactly the same. Betty Ford had chemo. Jean's mother did not. Betty Ford is still alive and Jean's mother died within five years. I was glad I decided to have chemo, even if it meant putting up with the fog.

Jane Shotkin, the oncology nurse, told me that people who do more cerebral kind of work have more trouble with chemo. That reassured me because I felt so unfocused. My office sent a list of addresses for me to review for a business mailing. I sat at the computer and literally cried as I tried to choose a dozen appropriate contacts from a list of over 100 possible names. I simply could not focus enough to make detailed decisions. Bob made me leave the computer and I later sent a message to the office, asking them to make the selection.

Howard described his fog:

> *I understand fully the issue of being in a fog during the chemo. I am just coming out of the round which ended a week ago. This last session has been the worst. I have two more to go. Ugh. I felt awful and could not think. I just stare off in space counting the hours*

until the situation passes. No one who has not gone though such an ordeal can understand it because words do not describe it. In any event, know you have an understanding and empathetic friend. Someday we shall celebrate the end of all of this.

I joked to friends that the lack of focus made me wonder if I had brain cancer rather than breast cancer. That was typical of the black humor that cancer patients are allowed to use with one another. Another laugh came when we heard news of a rumor that Bob had cancer. That originated with someone overhearing someone who repeated what someone else said, and so on, just like the old children's game of telephone. Since we were waiting to receive notification of Bob's next Army assignment, I hoped that the assignments office did not get wind of that misinformation.

Easter arrived within days of my third chemo treatment, and again Bob had planned a trip away from the site of my illness. Chris agreed that, during weeks one and three of each cycle, I could travel if I carried an antibiotic with me and promised to go immediately to a hospital if I had a fever. Ashley planned to spend Easter with her church youth group doing service projects in Ukraine. Bob and I did not want to spend Easter in our "sick house" without any of the girls there to celebrate with us.

On Good Friday, Ashley left at 4 a.m. I did not sleep much the night before, knowing we would rise early to get her on the way. During the night, I could feel the strength of the chemo coursing through my body as I lay awake in bed for hours. After Ashley's departure, I slept until 9 a.m. and then tried to prepare for the trip. The chemo fog and fatigue took over. I simply stood in the middle of the bedroom and cried, unable to choose items of clothing from the closet. Bob did nothing to rush me, and we eventually left at 1 p.m. with lunch in the car. For the first time, I had trouble riding and I felt pretty queasy, so I tried to sleep in the car.

We drove six hours to St. Lo, France, where we spent the night in a wonderful old French chateau with twenty sleeping rooms. The owner had been a *Tour de France* leader in the seventies and his bikes and awards, as well as World War II memorabilia, graced the chateau. We dined in a beautiful renovated stone farmhouse across the courtyard from the chateau, being served family style at a huge dining table with madame seated at the head.

On our first night, most of the guests were Brits and we enjoyed them, but we spoke French with madame. Before dessert, she gathered us all outside to see the Hale Bopp comet, spectacular with its long tail trailing behind. When Bob and I returned to our room and looked out of our windows, the brilliant stars in the night sky appeared to be within reach because there were no lights to hide the constellations.

On Saturday, we drove to Mont St. Michel, the monastery built on the pinnacle of a small rock island. While architecturally magnificent, it seemed far too touristy. When we arrived, I felt very shaky. Despite moderate temperatures, I shivered and my teeth chattered as we walked. We wandered on our own rather than take a two-hour tour which I could not have stood. We had a picnic lunch in the car and then drove to Bayeux. I slept most of the way in the car. There we viewed the Bayeux tapestry dating from the eleventh century, illustrating William the Conqueror's Battle of Hastings, after which he became king of Britain. Not at all what I expected, it presented a fascinating work of art and interesting history. But I did not have the stamina to study it. I needed a nap.

Again, dinner with madame at 7:30 p.m. and twice as many guests, mostly French. I sat next to a Belgian physician, exercising my French language skills. Ironic that we had made this trip to get away from the site of my sickness, and I dined with a Belgian doctor. He and his wife were there to look at the birds, so we talked about that, but I also told him briefly about my experience at Jules Bordet.

On Sunday, it did not seem at all like Easter. I missed the girls. We celebrate many family traditions at Easter. Even before having children, Bob and I would invite our friends to our home to dye Easter eggs, and the girls loved the tradition. Sadly, the Chateau did not have colored eggs for the continental breakfast, nor any other sign of Easter. When I felt low, all kinds of things seemed to be wrong. For example, I realized that only Bob's office knew our itinerary and it would be closed until Tuesday. I imagined terrible things happening to the girls or our families with no one able to reach us. Maybe that depression added to a difficult day.

We left the chateau and traveled the Normandy D-Day invasion route along the beaches. I did not feel well and spent much of the time sleeping in the car. Even at the U.S. cemetery at Omaha Beach, I slept in the car while Bob wandered around. When awake, I became nauseated and claustrophobic and I could not stand the wig. I wore a denim hat that came down low around my head to hide my baldness. As I reclined in the car, I could see myself in the side-view mirror, and I wondered if people thought

I was a dead body when they passed the car.

From Normandy, we drove to Cherbourg and took a five-hour ferry to Portsmouth. Our British navy friends met us and took us to their house high on the hills overlooking Portsmouth harbor. On Monday morning, Ed arranged for a special tour of Admiral Nelson's tall warship, HMS Victory, from the Battle of Trafalgar in the early 1800s. Although fascinating to see the four decks as they were originally used for living and fighting, I started feeling bad after only twenty minutes. Ed drove us home, but I had to ask him to stop the car because I was so nauseated. With a brand new Saab, he surely did not want me to throw up in it. The fresh air saved me, but it was embarrassing.

On Tuesday, we drove to Cardiff, Wales, to visit friends. The beautiful ride from Portsmouth through Bath to Cardiff passed through gorgeous countryside with many large stone manors, farms and rolling fields. The castles and ruins created a fairy tale impression. I slept on and off to ward off car sickness. After a pub lunch outside Bath, we made the final drive to Cardiff and I went straight to bed. The three days we spent there were relaxed and low stress, but peppered with more torturous and bizarre dreams. In fact, twice I awakened Bob in the middle of the night, calling out in my sleep. When that happened, I would be exhausted the next morning.

I wrote to Kennon describing several different dreams:

April 3, 1997

1. *I was in a place of violence and people were being attacked and killed. I didn't know anyone, but a woman was helping me. We tried to get away but found a bucket with a bloody arm in it. We retraced our steps. She said it was okay if a man named "Soso" would help us. But he wasn't there and she called to him. She was going to leave and I was terrified. I kept calling out—that was when I woke Bob up, crying, "Help."*

2. *I wanted to take a shower so I could go somewhere because I was late. Bob had been in the bathroom and locked the door. I wanted to get in. Finally, he got out and it was my turn. I couldn't get the door locked, and people kept coming in and out. I didn't want to get undressed and show I only had one breast. I kept trying to lock the door, but the lock was broken.*

109

Finally, I screamed, "What do I have to do to get any privacy?" That was the second time I woke Bob up, but my cries were incoherent.

3. *I was in Williamsburg staying at the Williamsburg Lodge, but I couldn't get there. I was with all these strange people who weren't my family. They were treating me like one of them, but I felt like I had to prove to them that I was normal and had a family who loved me. My hair was wet and kinky and I kept trying to hide it under a scarf (like I'm wearing a scarf now to hide my baldness). I needed to get checked in so I could go wherever I was supposed to be. The Colonial Williamsburg bus asked for my room key to assure I was reserved. I had to put the key in a keyhole on the back of the bus and I had trouble reaching it because I couldn't lift my arm on the surgery side high enough to turn it. A man helped me. The bus driver said to follow him, not asking me to get on. An older woman was with me (maybe Mother at that point), and we were having trouble keeping up. Then I realized where we were, but construction had changed things. There was a new building where I was teaching the management course that I used to teach when I worked at Arco Alaska. And another building that had something to do with my past, not sure what.*

4. *The day before, during my nap, I had a bizarre dream. I was in Williamsburg and wanted to get in touch with a guy I had dated as a student because I needed to make someone jealous—not clear who. He found me and we were overjoyed to see each other. We were going away together for the weekend. But then another girl was there and he wanted to be with her, so he dumped me for her.*

5. *I'm in a room with West Point friends. In real life, I haven't told them I have cancer. In the dream, I am explaining to them how hard it was for me to let them know I have cancer and they are hurt that I didn't tell them. When I awoke, a few hours later, the dream was so real that I had the sensation that I needed to tell Bob that I had seen our friends.*

This is all I can remember of several days of distorted dreams. As I did my shoulder exercises this morning, I got all teary and won-

dered if the murder dream where I yelled help was the death of my "former" life. Maybe that's too literal. I don't have energy now to work with my dreams, but I wanted to capture them before they fade too much.

Kennon responded immediately, again with helpful interpretations of the dreams. After the dream about our friends, I asked Bob's sister to let them know about the cancer. I also suggested that she tell everyone she thought might want to know. It relieved the pressure on me, as I had told my William and Mary friends, and brought me more prayers and positive thoughts from others.

The cumulative effect of the chemo had its wearing effects on our family and support group, too. Kennon wrote:

April 6, 1997

I just wanted to send you some cheer. CHEER! CHEER! CHEER!

I have thought so much about what you are feeling and what you wrote in your letter with your dreams. Today I went to the Jung Institute for a meeting with a friend who is going through breast cancer and chemo right now. It was the first time I had seen her since her surgery and when she walked in the room without a wig I immediately flashed on your telling me about waiting in the car for Bob with your hat on, wondering if people thought you were a dead body.

Soon after we started to talk, I started to cough and I couldn't stop and couldn't breathe. I knew that I was having an emotional reaction and that the feelings I hadn't expressed when I read your letter (just wanting to cry and come protect you) were coming out in the most inappropriate place.

I left the room, got water and stayed out until I was okay. I guess I just want to tell you that I am so angry and upset that you are having to go through this. It makes me want to "tell off" God.

On our return home, we had news from Andy and Lynne about his treatment. It had taken a month for all the consults and decisions, and he was glad to be moving forward. Andy likened his treatment to an infantry battle. Since I had invoked Saint Barbara, patron saint of the field artillery, this allowed the usual good-natured rivalry between an infantryman and an artilleryman. Andy wrote:

> *The special forces units have been sent in before the battle begins to start disrupting supply lines and to get the cancer to consolidate for the real battle.*
>
> *The radiation is to prep the battlefield and try to block the escape of any of the little cells as well as contain the area. After a couple weeks' rest I will go in for the seed implant. This will be outpatient treatment with the procedure lasting less than an hour and a couple more hours for recovery. I should be able to walk away (not ride a bike). Assuming I've done everything else right, and on time, I will have total victory (and no prisoners). (See Bob Glacel, it takes an infantryman, on the ground.).*
>
> *While the infantrymen are kicking butt I should have few side effects.*
>
> *Andy*

So, for both of us and so many others, the battle raged on.

You've Got Mail

We returned from our short trip to France and England just as the "danger" period began and my counts were dropping. Chris was concerned about my susceptibility to germs and kept me isolated except for physical therapy. Although I went to physical therapy three or four times a week, my shoulder continued to get worse and the pain was terrible. I have a friend, also a breast cancer survivor, who suffered bursitis in her shoulder some years after surgery and says that, without a doubt, the pain of the bursitis was much worse than the pain of either her mastectomy or reconstruction. In fact, she admits that, even though a good Roman Catholic, she wondered if she could continue living with such pain and wondered if ending her own life might be preferable.

Bob checked the mail daily because the prosthesis I had ordered should have arrived. If my counts were high enough to allow us to go to Portugal during the third week of the cycle, I needed the prosthesis to use in the bathing suit. The little cotton prosthesis that Madame Carstairs had made would never look right if I went in the water. Day after day, no package arrived. Again, I imposed on my friend Linda to check with the store where we had bought it. I had paid for it to be express mailed to the Army Post Office (APO) which should have taken three days. The store records showed it had been sent three weeks before. Obviously something had gone wrong, but the mail room manager was less than helpful, telling Linda that he knew his business and knew how to ship to an APO.

During the week of my isolation, Ashley's school had their annual scholarship fund auction. We had attended the year before and had such fun, as well as coming home with a myriad of interesting things donated from different NATO nations. Ashley worked at the auction, and I wanted to see the auction items so she could bid for us if she wanted. I knew I couldn't stay around so many people, but I went inside when we delivered Ashley just so I could look. I kept my hands in my coat pockets, hoping that people wouldn't offer to shake hands, which all Europeans do. Many people were surprised and pleased to see me since I had not been in much evidence in recent months. One lovely woman ran over to hug me, and I jumped back and exclaimed, "Don't touch me!" I realized later how rude that was. I had become absolutely paranoid about germs.

Ashley would agree with that. On more than one occasion, I had begged Chris not to hospitalize me when my counts were low, promising to stay at home with just Bob, Ashley, and the poodle. Ashley had enough opportunity to bring germs home from school. I would not allow her to visit her friends or have friends over to the house if there were the least hint that they might have a cold. On one afternoon, I took Ashley to the medical clinic for an appointment, and I wore a mask. As we entered the lobby, she saw her best friend. Darci had missed nearly a week of school with some kind of bug that had not yet been diagnosed. To my horror, Ashley started to run to give Darci a hug. I grabbed her and literally dragged her away kicking and screaming, and I doubt that either girl ever quite accepted that I believed my action to be justified.

By day fifteen, Chris determined that my counts were high enough that Bob and I could go to Portugal for four days before my final chemo treatment. We flew on a charter to Lisbon, changing planes for a hop to the Algarve on the south coast. In the Lisbon airport, Bob left me momentarily to find a *Herald Tribune* newspaper. I begged him to hurry back and not leave me for too long. I had the feeling that, without him, something would surely go wrong. I had traveled all over the world by myself, and this was a new and unsettling feeling. Even Bob commented that I did not seem the same person. The real difference seemed to be in risk-taking. I simply wanted things decided for me.

The four days in Portugal were great for Bob. He had been working so hard to take care of me, to keep up at work, and to deal with his own emotional reactions. He faced two solid months of travel starting in early May, and he needed a break before that routine began. He played golf every day. On the first day, I went with him and rode in the cart, with great discomfort. My eyes felt dry and gritty from the chemo. I had lost most of my eyelashes and the sand blew dust into my eyes, so I was in pain until I could get my contact lenses out. Then I would be afraid that the wind would blow the contact away. The chemo made me very susceptible to the sun, so I used heavy sunscreen and wore long sleeves and a hat over my wig. My shoulder ached terribly, and I could not find a comfortable position in the small golf cart.

After that first day, I stayed in our condo while Bob golfed. I walked around the garden or sat in the shade by the pool. I could not go in the pool since I had no prosthesis to use in the bathing suit. I napped in the afternoon, and on one afternoon I actually rewrote an article that VIMA submitted for publication. To accomplish something energized me more than anything else had in a long time.

On our last day, we did some sightseeing and a little shopping. If only I had felt better, we could have done major damage to the credit card. We wandered through the fish market, the open market, the pottery market. We drove along country roads that featured lovely little white-washed villages. But, again, the car sickness hit me, and at one point, Bob had to pull over for me to be sick. All I wanted was to get home and go to bed.

As I faced my final chemo treatment, Howard finished his fourth out of six. His was very different than mine. He received an injection every day for five days and then had three weeks off. His side effects were also very different. Kennon wrote:

> *Howard just finished his fourth chemo treatment and is feeling bad. He said yesterday that if the cancer comes back he will not go through chemo again. His insides burn, he cannot sleep, he cannot focus or think or remember, and he gets depressed, which his oncologist said is part of these particular drugs. Tonight while I was fixing dinner he showed me his feet that are full of blisters and cracked ever so deeply from the chemo. I said to him that I feel so badly for him and I hope that I never have to go through the same thing. He started crying, saying that it is so horrible. His mouth is full of sores, he does not sleep at night, he feels like his insides are sloughing off and he is miserable. It is terrible to watch and I feel helpless. I feel so awful for both of you.*
>
> *Today as Howard drove downtown, I felt the car slowing down several times, almost halting. Finally I realized that Howard was*

simply forgetting what he was doing. When we got downtown, he suddenly stopped the car and I asked him why. He said, "It's a crosswalk and these women want to cross." Well, yes there were women wanting to cross but the rush hour traffic was speeding by in all the other lanes. Then he decided to go and almost ran over a man trying to cross the street legally at the light. We laughed, but it is so sad. This chemotherapy is just awful.

I could identify with Howard. Even though I knew that this was my last chemo treatment, I dreaded going to Jules Bordet. Just going into the dreary building and seeing so many very sick people made me queasy. I had so much more nausea this time, throughout the whole three weeks. When I told that to Dr. Kenton, he just laughed and said that nausea after the first three days was not chemo-induced. Maybe not physically, I thought to myself, but certainly psychologically. I wished so much for an oncologist who would deal with me as a person. Sometimes I wondered if Dr. Kenton remembered me from one visit to the next.

I was also very tired of being a pin cushion. Always, it took two or three sticks to draw blood and two or three sticks to insert the IV for the chemo. Usually they had to resort to using tiny veins in the back of my hand or in my wrist. Anticipating all of this, I donned my red outfit spiritlessly and went to Bordet for my last chemo treatment. Even with all the symbols in my pockets, I felt lifeless.

The fourth and final treatment of chemotherapy was truly the worst one. With every visit to the oncologist, he would read through a longer list of possible side effects to see if I had suffered any of them. Since the effects of chemo were cumulative, I seemed to be having more. At this last visit, he gave me more anti-nausea medication. I had a couple of sores in my mouth, but they were not too bad. My skin was very dry and my eyes felt very gritty.

My counts had not recovered and were dangerously low for another chemo treatment. However, Dr. Kenton said he "closed his eyes" to the counts for my last treatment. On the one hand, I was glad to get it over with. On the other hand, I wished we had stayed in Portugal and voluntarily delayed the treatment even without knowing what the counts would be. In retrospect, I wonder if it weren't highly irresponsible for Dr. Kenton to allow me to receive the treatment. With each treatment, the counts were lower than before and he never provided anything to stimulate reproduction of the blood cells. So both physically and mentally, I felt worse and became more isolated.

During this visit, I begged him to do something about my shoulder. It had become truly excruciating and I could not bear anyone to touch it. The pain interrupted my sleep many times each night, and this made me more tired, more emotional, and less able to cope. The physical therapy was so painful that I cried through the stretching. Dr. Kenton ordered an x-ray and an ultrasound and he assured me that a new malignancy did not cause the pain. What he meant as reassurance truly startled me. Somehow I did not realize at that time that a cancer patient must forever be concerned about chronic pain as it might indicate a metastasis.

All of this combined—the shoulder, the chemo, the low cell counts, not to mention the cancer—put me in a precarious psychological state. Not only was I unable to accomplish what I could before cancer, but I also felt that I had become less of a whole person. Feeling this way, I began to have trouble turning things around to look at the positive. What I needed to do was to learn to let go and let life flow around me. A friend suggested that I...

> *...just relax in the arms of caring thoughts of those who love you and let it go. You don't have to control, to entertain, to be responsive, to manage, to lead all the time. You need to give that up periodically and just give in. Some would say to a superior being—others would say to those who care about you. We both need to realize what a gift we are giving people when we do that.*

The night of my fourth and last treatment was the worst night I had from the chemo. Even though I took Tylenol P.M., I awoke feeling a heat going through my body. It actually seemed as though I could feel the chemo bubbling through my veins. The liquids were cold when they went into my body, but this was a radiating heat. My head throbbed and my ears rang. The next morning I awoke with a red flush all over my face. It was as if the red toxin were coming out of my pores. I felt hot to the touch, but did not have a fever.

Ashley and I had watched a video on chemo. Much to my surprise, it said that for every month of chemo, one can expect two months of recovery. I had figured that by mid-May, after day twenty-two of this final cycle, I would begin to feel fine. With this new information, it seemed as though it might be Thanksgiving before I would have the stamina to work the way I used to. That projection disappointed me, but thankfully, the chemo treatments were finished.

After we returned from Portugal and there was no more urgency, the prosthesis finally arrived. The whole scene added some levity to an otherwise depressing time. The manager of the store's mail room who had defensively retorted that he knew how to ship to an APO obviously did not. While he had used the APO address on the box, he wrote BELGIUM in large letters at the bottom and must have thrown it into the international mail sack. He also had not filled out the proper customs paperwork for international shipping. When it arrived through the usually very slow Belgian post office, they delivered it to the Army mail room in the NATO military headquarters building.

Without customs forms identifying the contents of the box, the Army mail room would not accept it without opening it. When I imagined these young soldiers opening a box and staring at a fake breast, all I could do was laugh. Most women my age have not seen a prosthesis, but these young hormone-charged soldiers must have been incredulous. It was worth the wait to get a chuckle when I needed it. And after seeing what it was, they had to call me to say, "You've got mail."

The Bottom of the Barrel

Although the chemo ended, healing did not. I realized that cancer is a long-term illness. When the diagnosis is new, people rally around and the support is incredible. As the illness goes on and on, others understandably get on with their lives. And, of course, when the patient feels well enough to be out, then others see her looking her best. At other times, she doesn't feel like going out, so others do not see the down times.

A friend from the States asked, "I wonder if it's too hard for a friend of a lower rank to just help the general's wife." I imagined that to be true. People were kind if I ran into them in the clinic, and they asked how I felt. But few offered other support, encouragement, or assistance. I called an American wife admitted to Bordet for leukemia, and she apologized for never having called me, saying she thought it inappropriate to call the general's wife. Added to that, we lived in a Belgian neighborhood with no one who said more than "*Bonjour*" as we walked the dog, or who occasionally waved to us over the fence. Some of them didn't even do that. I had talked several times to the woman who lived across the backyard from us, but often when we came outside, her family would go inside.

Rhonda described the current situation when she wrote:

> *Don't be surprised if you go through a letdown, or feelings of anxiety or depression when the chemo is over. Your friends and family will not be so attentive. People will assume that you are okay, and will no longer give any special treatment. You will get on with your life. Nevertheless, the fear is something that you will have to learn to live with. I do experience dread when I have my six month check-*

ups with the oncologist or my surgeon, or when I have my mammo-
gram. Last summer when I had lost all the weight and had ab-
dominal pain and then a question about my liver on the CT scan,
I was terrified. I felt much more lonely and fearful of these things
than I did with the surgery and chemotherapy when everyone was
hovering.

I've just violated my cardinal rule, namely to never tell horror
stories to someone who is sick. Moreover, I've just reread the way I
stated it, and I realize that it sounds as if I'm presuming to tell you
how you will feel or how your friends and family will react. I'm just
telling you how I felt and how I felt my friends and family were
reacting, which may not be an accurate portrayal of how they were
actually feeling about me. Part of my problem is that I apparently
always convey that my life is under control and that I don't need
any help.

Without the support of Americans and with the understandable cultural reticence of many of the Europeans, I felt starved for contact. My e-
mail support group seemed my best contact with those who would love
and support me, but they couldn't touch me. I continued to hear from
more friends in the States, some of them long-term friends. I wished so
much that these friends were here with me in Belgium. It would have been
a very different experience, and much less lonely. Knowing how much the
American military on U.S.-run bases takes care of its own, a friend wrote:

I hope all the other military wives there smothered you with love,
prayers and support while you were going through all the chemo.

That made me feel even sorrier for myself, thinking of what I had missed
with my friends being so far away.

Chris continued to worry about my counts dropping since Dr. Kenton
had given me the chemo without recovery of my white cells and neutro-
phils. He cautioned me not to go anywhere except to physical therapy, to
wear a mask there, and to even wear a mask at home. That got old fast.

On April 30, I had another cultural experience. Scheduled for a shoulder x-ray and ultrasound at Jules Bordet, and knowing that drapes are
nonexistent in Belgian hospitals, I took a small sterile towel with me. I

undressed in the dressing room, held the towel under both arms across my chest, and walked out to the x-ray room. The x-ray technician placed me in front of the machine, quickly pulled the towel away from me, and said *"Ce n'est pas necessaire"* as she threw it across the room onto a table. There I stood, bare-chested, lop-sided with a single breast, and scarred, as she took eight different x-rays in different positions. Meanwhile, people wandered in and out of the room and past the open door with me in full view. Honestly, there was no such thing as modesty in Belgian hospitals.

As I understood the French, they decided I had acute tendinitis and should stop physical therapy for a few weeks. Dr. Kenton would have a full report for me. By the time he called me to his office, x-ray had closed for the day. The next day, May 1, was a holiday. He said he would get a full report on Friday and call me. He told me that after day fifteen, when my blood count should start climbing, I could resume the anti-inflammatory medication, and that I should continue to rub a medicated gel on my shoulder.

I reported these results to Chris and had blood work done in Mons. My counts again were dangerously low, and so the isolation continued. Bob was scheduled to begin his two months of travel soon, and I felt so alone and very weepy. Without him, I felt rudderless as we navigated each day. At the same time, we learned that our next assignment would be in Fort Hood, Texas. We did not know anything about Fort Hood or about the command Bob would assume. But with a definite location, we had to prepare for the move, and the whole idea exhausted me. The movers would come in early June, and Bob's travel schedule consumed most of May and June. I did not know how I would ever manage all this by myself.

I had written little e-mail, and my mother wrote with concern. My feelings of listlessness were obvious in my response:

> *Hi Mom,*
> *I had a terrible night last night. I woke up almost crying with the pain in my shoulder. I took Tylenol 3 and slept until about 4 a.m., then was awake from that point on. Other than that, I feel a little better today. Bob and I have been going through one room at a time getting ready for the movers. I took a nap this afternoon.*

Five days after the shoulder x-ray, we still had not heard from Dr. Kenton. Marie tried repeatedly to call him for me. I e-mailed Dr. Diehl asking his advice about whether to continue physical therapy. The x-ray technician thought that physical therapy might be making the shoulder worse, but the physical therapist thought that if we stopped therapy the shoulder could completely freeze. The surgical treatment to unfreeze a shoulder did not sound pretty. Marie also believed that there was more to deal with than tendinitis, because my range of motion had decreased since the first month after surgery.

Finally, Marie reached Dr. Kenton who still had not looked at either the x-rays or the ultrasound. Marie held the phone while he called radiology for the report. The x-rays showed nothing irregular. The ultrasound showed acute tendinitis and something wrong with the rotator cuff to indicate a frozen shoulder. Dr. Kenton suggested I see a rheumatologist or orthopedic surgeon. Marie knew a good orthopedic surgeon in Brussels whom she wanted me to see, but I had no energy to do that. Tired of trips to Brussels to see doctors and with Bob away, I could not begin to imagine finding a new address by myself. Marie kindly offered to take a day of leave to drive me to Brussels. However, Chris thought I might see improvement in the next few weeks as the chemo left my body and my counts started to rise, allowing healing in my shoulder to begin. We decided to wait for two weeks before making an appointment.

Along with everything else, Murphy's Law seemed to be firmly in effect in Belgium. Bob departed on May 3 for the first leg of his two month tour around the NATO member nations. On Monday morning, the garage door wouldn't open so I could not get the car out to go to physical therapy. Three workmen spent all afternoon working on that. The night before, we had endured very hard spring rains, and the basement had flooded. Workmen discovered a hole in the wall where the water was coming in. Unfortunately, this made it the landlord's problem, not the Army's. The workmen were thrilled not to have to deal with it, but I was used to the landlord's nonreaction to house problems, so I was unhappy. It remained my problem. The water had gotten a bag of charcoal wet, and in moving it, the bag broke leaving wet black charcoal all over the floor. I left it there, hoping it would go away by itself.

Kennon wrote:

May 7, 1997
Oh my god, what a terrible situation for you. Doesn't all of this
make you think, "Well, it is clear I am not in control of my life,

nor my health although I work hard at it, nor my relationships as Bob goes off for two months, nor my physical property as the basement floods. Therefore, I will simply lay back a bit and get sure about myself, that's all I can do." I only say this because it is the philosophy I applied to myself after feeling so awful the other day. Now I feel better. Howard realized that he was freaking out over his chemotherapy, and I realized that I was doing the best I could. Both of us realized that life is bigger than both of us. How are you and Ashley doing?

The good news was that Ashley and I were doing great together. She became such a joy and a support to me, and I knew that with Bob gone, I could not make it without her. I felt the need of family so much, and I could hardly wait for Jenn to come home in mid-May and Sarah in June. During evenings when Ashley and I were alone, we often watched old home videos together. There were times that we laughed until we cried, reminding me of Norman Cousins who "laughed himself well." I needed that laughter the most now when I was at rock bottom.

I summed it up for Linda:

May 8, 1997

Thanks for your long, newsy note. Maybe it will snap me out of my lethargy enough to write to you I'm just not feeling very chatty these days. The fourth (and final, thank God) chemo hit me much harder than the previous ones. It has been three weeks ago yesterday, so healing should be commencing about now. But, I feel that I have a long way to go, both physically and mentally. I'm lethargic, and very fragile ego-wise.

The chemo cycle officially ended on May 8. Stupidly, I had thought that I would immediately feel better. But that just was not the case. The chemicals had dragged my body down to a very low point physically and my mind to a state of depression. It would actually take a long time to get back to normal. For five months, I had been mostly "out of sight," and so it felt as though I were also "out of mind" and very alone.

Part Three
Hope

Hope is contagious

and it can metastasize

faster than cancer cells.

—*Bob Stone*

Jenny Stone Humphries

Coming Up for Air

Entering and emerging from the spell of the chemo seemed a gradual process, unlike the immediate effect of the surgery that had felt as though I had run into a wall at breakneck speed. I had gone on disability from VIMA and had told Provident insurance company that after completing chemotherapy in May, I planned to go back to work. Provident did not pressure me in the least. They only required monthly paperwork describing my daily schedule with a doctor's verification of my current medical state. That was not a problem. I still endured physical therapy three days a week, napped in the afternoons, and had trouble focusing.

I had tried throughout the treatment to keep up with business issues at VIMA, particularly the financials, but the chemo fog made it difficult to concentrate. While I tried to offer business support, it was clear that there were things I could not do. I did not have enough stamina to get through a day with a client, or a week's seminar, or to travel to our clients. While my blood counts had regenerated enough that I did not have to be isolated, it took a long time for them to regain the normal range. And it also took time for me to regain the ability to focus on detail without feeling very stressed. We had begun work on a new corporate brochure a few months before I was diagnosed. I simply could not find the energy to work with the marketing consultant to answer questions about our work, to look at paper samples, or to proofread pages.

As I came out of the fog, often I would learn of something that I had heard or something that had happened during the previous three months, yet I would have no real recollection. Months later when I visited Williamsburg, I happily noted that a manager at the Alumni Society was pregnant. I congratulated her over the wonderful news, only to be re-minded that I had congratulated her back in March and had sent e-mail good wishes too. I did not remember any of that.

With Bob gone, Ashley had become very protective of me. Once she accepted the role of being the only daughter at home to care for Mom, she took it seriously. In one instance, she had a long-term substitute in a class at school who had not been trained as a teacher and was not very effective in the classroom. One day when Ashley challenged him, he retorted with a sarcastic remark about whether she might get her mother to come take up for her. He probably did not know about my condition; it was just a remark to put Ashley in her place. Ashley, however, took it as a direct attack on me. Already being attacked by cancer, I did not need to be attacked by her sub-stitute teacher. She grabbed all her books and ran crying from the room, swearing she would never go back into the class as long as he was there.

We shared some good talks during the time that Bob was away. One day, she said, "You know, Mom, losing your hair wasn't so bad after all."

I started to explain to her that it felt pretty bad to me, when I realized she was telling me that her worst fears about having a bald mom had not panned out.

No longer in medical isolation, I began to get out more. I even bought lots of red geraniums and planted our flower boxes. One day as I drove to the Mons Grand Place, I realized that the last time I had been there was at the Christmas Market with Bob and Jenn, just two days after my diagno-sis. As I drove home, I started crying. It felt as though I had lost five months of my life. We loved living in Europe so much, and we were leav-ing without having done many things we wanted to do. I sent Bob an e-mail to tell him that, and I admitted:

May 15, 1997
And, despite all your good assurances, I'm still feeling quite shaky about my attractiveness to you. Sorry to bring that up, but I still live with it constantly and it helps me to share it. After all, you're my best friend and maybe you can help me feel better.

Bob returned briefly to Mons on May 17, arriving on the same plane that brought Jenn home from college. They found me still in bed when they arrived at the house. Our poodle, Souci, was so excited to see them that she peed all over the kitchen floor. Bob cleaned that up, and Jenn came upstairs to find me with an ice pack on my shoulder. Then, Bob let Souci run upstairs and her excitement got the better of her again, so she peed all over the bedspread, sheets, and me. It was not an auspicious start to the day, but what could we do? We laughed.

At that point, with my family back home, I saw a clear turnaround in the direction of my emotional health. The emotional recovery presented more of a challenge than I had bargained for, but being surrounded by family, made it easier to bear. Within a few days of Jenn's arrival, Howard and Kennon's son, Colin, and his friend arrived from France. With a house full of teenagers, I found it difficult to be as self-focused as I had been for the three months of isolation. Colin had not seen his father since December, following Howard's surgery for colon cancer. I promised Kennon that I would talk to Colin about the effects of the chemo, and it occurred to me that I should probably have the same talk with Jenn. I wrote to Kennon:

May 21, 1997

It's the end of the afternoon, and we've had a wonderful day with Colin and James. They are so nice and easygoing and helpful that it has given me energy today. Bob left early for two days in Germany, Ashley left for school, and Colin was the first one of the kids to get up. He and I ended up sitting over about a two-hour breakfast and just talking. We talked a lot about his year in France and Sarah's year in Russia, but we also talked a lot about cancer. He wanted to know how it felt to have cancer and to face the future. He's trying to relate to what he has missed with you, Howard.

I was very honest with him from my perspective and pretty detailed about breast cancer—probably more than he ever wanted to know. But he had good questions, talked about how badly he felt that he wasn't at home to go through this with both of you, and how much he wants to be home now. He wants to spend time with you, Howard, and to take some of the load off of you, Kennon. I warned him about the chemo fog, the lack of patience, the sometimes illogical emotions, and the physical and emotional effects I feel. I hope it will help him be prepared to come home at the end of Howard's chemo cycle. He talked about how hard it is to see one's parent ill, the person who has always been so strong and steady. I hope you'll all be able to talk a lot about how you're feeling when he comes home, because he seems to want that.

Physical therapy continued, and that was the one thing dragging me down. My shoulder was so painful. Chris took me off the anti-inflammatory drug because he said it should not be taken long-term. On the recommendation of the therapist at Bethesda Naval Hospital, Marie had changed my treatment to electro-therapy followed by lots of stretching in all directions, and then ice massage. My shoulder always felt so painful after the stretching that the ice massage felt good. Marie's fingers would get so cold, and I just wanted her to continue cooling down my shoulder.

She fitted me for a portable TENS unit with electrodes attached to the front and back of my shoulder. I wore a little box on my belt from which I could regulate the intensity and pattern of electrical stimulus that went into the tendons and soft tissue. It helped tremendously to decrease the pain, but did not increase my mobility.

In late May, I accompanied Bob on his NATO trip to Norway and Denmark. I had lived in Norway as an exchange student in 1966 when my Norwegian family had accepted me as their daughter. I felt very close to them. *Mor* could express herself in writing so beautifully, and she had been distraught at the news that her "other" daughter had been stricken with cancer. She had written frequently during the previous months. *Far* had been my surrogate father for thirty-one years since my own Dad had died when I was only eleven. Having the chance to be back in their home as I healed was so special. They loved me unconditionally, as only parents can, and we could be perfectly natural together.

Our departure from Brussels seemed uneventful until I discovered that the TENS unit set off the airport security detectors. Trying to explain in fractured French what I was wearing, I wondered if it looked like a bomb.

I stayed four days with *Mor* and *Far* at their summer house on an island in the Oslo fjord. *Mor* and I took walks in nature, and I felt better just by being surrounded by loving Norwegian "parents." From there, Bob and I flew to Copenhagen and spent a day with Danish friends. We celebrated our friend Jeanne's birthday in Tivoli, Copenhagen's famous amusement park. While Bob worked, I went with Jeanne and Benn to the north coast to Hamlet's castle. I remembered taking that route by bicycle back in 1966 and wondered how I ever made it.

On our return to Mons, Bob spent five days at home helping while the packers prepared to ship our household goods to Texas. The week's schedule was exhausting, with Ashley's National Honor Society induction, two farewell dinners for Bob and me, an appointment at Jules Bordet, and the packers for four days. That's the kind of schedule that we were used to pre-cancer, and I optimistically thought that I did not have time to feel sick anymore.

Suddenly, it seemed as if someone tapped me on the shoulder and said, "Not so fast, Barbara." After a rushed trip to Bordet, during which the doctor was running late so we never saw her, causing a late arrival back for Ashley's Honor Society induction, we went to dinner. During the meal, I felt so terrible that I left the restaurant and lay down in the back seat of the car. That was a reminder that I needed to continue to rest in order to fully recover from the chemotherapy.

Bob left again, this time to Rome, and Jenn accompanied me to Brussels for medical appointments. I had finally allowed Marie to book an appointment with an orthopedic surgeon because I did not see much improvement in my shoulder. The TENS unit reduced some pain, but I still lost sleep. Marie did not see a lot of improvement in range of motion. Dr. Sepulchre found that when flexion of my arm reached thirty degrees, the scapula moved and caused complete cessation of rotation. He injected my shoulder with prednisone. When the needle was inserted, liquid squirted out of the tissue. He concluded that I had bursitis and intraarticular effusion. Therefore, he suggested we continue with the same therapy. He believed that if I had continuous therapy, I could regain full range of motion in eighteen months to two years.

Jenn took me to Bordet to see Dr. Hertens one last time. She talked to Jenn about health implications for the daughter of a breast cancer patient. Spending a lot of time with me, she answered all my questions. I felt a real reluctance to leave her. The prospect of finding all new medical care providers seemed daunting. I owed my life to Dr. Hertens, and I fervently hoped that I would see her again some day.

After the appointment, Jenn and I met Christine for a last visit, a chance for a quick good-bye in person before we returned to the States. Christine was still having chemotherapy for the tumor on her liver, but she had bravely taken on a project of creating computer-generated original greeting cards that sold in the Bordet gift shop, raising money for the Institute. She proudly showed me some cards.

"I'm so sad to be leaving Belgium," I told her. "I feel as though I have lost five months of my life."

She gently chided me, reminding me of all the things that I had done during this time: found new friends, received the love and support of my e-mail buddies, friends, and family, reached out to others in need, traveled, and grown to be a different person.

She was right, and shortly thereafter, I woke up to a day when I realized I had come up from the depths. I wrote to my cousin, Jim:

> *With the increased activity around here, I haven't had much time to be sick, and I suddenly realized yesterday that I don't FEEL sick any more. Instead of feeling sick and having some good days, I feel pretty normal with some tired days. That's an enormous psychological turnaround for which I am grateful.*

As I climbed back up, it was only then that I realized how low I had been.

Au Revoir

The last few weeks in Belgium were both a sad time and a fun time. Happily, I felt better and could enjoy them. Several very special visitors came to Mons. Bodil, my Norwegian "sister" from my exchange student days, brought her daughter, Anine. During a long weekend together, we did a little sightseeing in the region. Although Bodil and I did not see each other often, we had a strong bond of sharing her parents, of visits on both sides of the ocean, and of children near the same age. Just a month before my diagnosis, we had rendezvoused in Oslo. She and I had slept in the same room and had reverted to our teenage behavior of giggling after we turned the lights out, each remembering more things to talk about as the night wore on. That November visit had actually made my subsequent diagnosis more poignant for my whole Norwegian family. They had been a big support on this side of the Atlantic.

Another long-time friend visited from France. Diddy had been my department chair on the faculty at the University of Alaska some thirteen years before. Our busy lives kept us from communicating often enough. Spending a semester with her daughter and a group of students in France, she was late to hear of my cancer. When she received the news, she immediately called. Over one weekend, she traveled by overnight train to Mons, spent a whole day with me, and then took another overnight train back to her students in southern France. We spent six hours sitting at an outdoor café. Only in Europe could we do that without pressure to leave. We ate lunch, coffee, dessert, and wine and talked for hours. It was a wonderful reunion and a special tribute to our friendship.

On June 28, Sarah returned home from her ten months in Russia, during which time she had not come home at all. She had had a difficult but wonderful year in Lomonosov, near Saint Petersburg. Her exchange family loved her as a daughter and sister, and she hated to leave them, but she wanted to see for herself that I was doing better. It had been hard on both of us to be apart for the entire time of my illness. Bob happened to be home for twenty-four hours, so he, Jenn, Ashley, and I gathered up Becky, Randy, and their son, Pete, to go to the airport. We weren't sure we would recognize Sarah. She had left Belgium with long curly hair, but she wrote that she had cut it very short. We knew that it had been several different colors during her stay in Russia, so who knew what it would look like?

Finally, she came through the doors of the customs hall, very thin in a tie-dyed T-shirt, with short, orangish hair. I reached her first, and we hugged and cried, until finally someone else asked for their turn to greet her. On the ride home, she talked nonstop.

Unfortunately, Bob departed for Greece the next morning, so we were a complete family for less than a day. In a few days, Ashley left for the United States. Sarah and Jenn both had lots of questions about what the previous five months had been like. We talked a lot about cancer and one morning, I said, "Do you want to see my scar?" I wanted to get beyond any fear they might have of walking in on me undressed and being embarrassed. Sarah immediately said yes, so I showed them the mastectomy incision. By this time, it had healed enough that it wasn't frightening, and I think it helped them both to know that, while it looked unusual, it was not terribly ugly.

Jenn was the next one to leave for the United States, going back for an internship on Capitol Hill. Sarah had only a few more days to adjust, pack for the move, and then depart for Greece to visit her best high school friend, the daughter of a Greek Air Force officer. Bob and I had a few more days to wind down and say good-bye to Belgium.

There were several dinners, parties, luncheons, and farewells for us and for others who were moving that summer. Because I had not seen many people for the previous five months, it provided a nice opportunity to reacquaint as well as to say the formal good-bye. Many of the wonderful NATO ladies who had been afraid to invade my privacy during the time of my treatment were so gracious. I could see in their eyes that they were glad to see me looking well again. Some of them probably did not even know I was wearing a wig because they had not seen me in so long. My German friend, Heide, confessed that she had been so worried about me and had been afraid to call. Her English was better than my German, but she was always embarrassed to use it. And speaking a foreign language over the phone is even more difficult than in person. She apologized for not being in touch.

At one farewell party, I spoke about the wives of three officers leaving Bob's branch. I thanked them for their support to me while I was ill and cited the specific kindness of two of them. After the remarks, the third wife came to me and cried.

"I wanted so much to help you, but I was scared," she confessed. "We are so alike in age and with children. It made me fear I could have cancer too."

The hardest good-bye was to Chris Georgantopoulos. To him, even more than Dr. Hertens, I owed my life. He had prescribed the original mammogram seven months before. He had been able to hold me throughout the treatment, as Jim Hines said a good doctor should do. He cared for all five of us at one time or another, always accessible, kind, competent, and going well beyond the call of duty. I knew I would never find another Chris Georgantopoulos, and I got very teary as I told him good-bye.

The support group was a farewell of thanks for all they had done for me and we had done for each other. The women had come together in support of one another even though the medical community did not sponsor a support group. We had given each other what was just as important—the ability to laugh at ourselves and the proof that there is life after cancer. Jane was already planning a black tie Breast Cancer Ball for September in order to raise funds for breast cancer research in Britain. I wished I could attend, but we were headed to the land of the Texas Two Step and blue jeans.

Bob and I spent our last two nights in a gorgeous chateau. We ate our last dinner at the same restaurant on the *Grand Place* where we had eaten our first dinner two years earlier. We said good-bye to the special friends who had been such a support in Mons, Paul and Janine, Liz and Peter. Almost seven months to the day from the mammogram that changed our lives, we bid *au revoir* to the site where I had been sick.

Deep in the Heart of Texas

Our first welcome back to the States came even before we reached Texas. Linda planned a dinner for us, inviting our close friends and family. The first time these members of my support group had seen me in the flesh since before cancer proved to be a wonderful reunion.

On July 18, Bob and Ashley and I flew to Texas and discovered our new home at Fort Hood. My overwhelming impression was HOT. I knew I would not be able to stand the wig for very long. I now had enough hair to wash, but not enough to go wigless. I didn't think the buzz-cut quite fit my personality.

Coming to a new Army post as a commander is a big deal. We were welcomed warmly, escorted everywhere, given tours, and hosted in people's homes for dinner. Everyone treated us with warmth and graciousness. While folks had been told that I was recovering from cancer, that was not something easily discussed on a first meeting. At Bob's change of command, we sat outside in the direct sun for well over an hour during the ceremony and speeches. I roasted with the wig on and worried about my exposed arm in the sunlight even though I had used sunscreen. After the ceremony, we greeted over 300 guests in a receiving line. Then I went home to bed.

The wives hosted a special welcome for me, and I decided to break the ice about the topic everyone seemed to be avoiding. After my introduction and the presentation of a gift, I spoke to all the ladies in attendance.

"I should probably warn you that if you think you see a less physically fit Demi Moore in the neighborhood, it is not the real G.I. Jane, but me without my wig."

Their laughter made the unspeakable a topic that we could address.

"I am happy to talk about my recovery from cancer, and happy to be in Texas where I can resume activities that have been on hold for these past seven months," I told them.

That evening, I met another club member who had recovered from breast cancer just a year before. I learned that club members were everywhere.

Not only the wig gave me problems in the heat of Texas. I had to be careful with what I wore when we were going to be out-of-doors, especially for a long period of time. One night we went to an outdoor picnic at the home of friends. We had known our hosts for many years and our daughters were best friends, but we did not know most of the other guests since we were new to Fort Hood. Obviously they did not know I had cancer and there was no reason to bring it up. It became apparent, though, that something strange was happening to my body when I looked down at my silk blouse and noticed a wet ring of perspiration surrounding the prosthesis. How embarrassing. How long, I wondered, had I been meeting new people with this wet circle over my nonexistent breast.

I made my immediate goal reestablishing medical care, which proved to be more difficult that I expected. During the two years since we had left the United States, the military had implemented a new health care system similar to a health management organization, managed by a civilian contractor. Apparently this was part of the failed national health care plan. Changes in the military medical care without the accompanying national health care system made it like a spoke without a wheel to support it.

I had been without physical therapy since July 10, and I could feel my shoulder stiffening and range of motion deteriorating despite the exercises I did daily at home. I had returned the portable TENS unit to the clinic in Belgium, and I needed another one from the medical facility at Fort Hood. I had carried my two-inch-thick medical records by hand from Belgium, having every document translated into English before I departed. Despite all the documentation, however, the system required that I start all over with a primary care provider in order to get consults written to the myriad of specialists whom I needed to see.

There could be as much as a thirty-day wait for a chronic illness and then an additional thirty-day wait for a consult with a specialist. I was not willing to wait for a problem that needed immediate and ongoing attention. Little did I know then that my effort to get access to quality care would ultimately lead me to the committee rooms of the Rayburn House

Office Building in Washington, D.C., where I would testify before a congressional committee. The nightmare began.

Because Bob pulled strings, an internist agreed to see me within two weeks. She did not take cancer lightly, and she understood that I was still very much in the recovery mode. I had not seen an oncologist for four months and should be having appointments quarterly during the first year. The doctor wrote a consult for oncology, but she also made sure that I was on the top of the list to see the visiting oncologist who only came to Fort Hood one day a month. Had we waited for the system to work, I might not see an oncologist for several more months. I shook my head, wondering if anyone ever joked about needing to see an oncologist. I didn't think so. I wondered why the official system made it so hard.

Physical therapy presented another issue. The physical therapy clinic in the Army hospital did not treat family members. Willing to go to a civilian provider, I requested a referral, a process that proved to be unwieldy. Following the doctor's advice, I walked my referral request through the system. That required carrying the paperwork between three separate buildings, waiting in lines at each place, getting a stamp on a piece of paper, being checked by two computer systems that did not talk to each other, and finally receiving a referral for an appointment. In the August heat, wearing a wig, recovering from chemotherapy, I was exhausted when I reached the final office.

"I can book an appointment for you next month," the health care finder told me.

"That's completely unacceptable!" I could hear my voice rising as I explained, "I have not had physical therapy for three weeks and I am losing mobility. I'm supposed to have continuous care."

The earliest available appointment was two weeks later, at which time I had been out of treatment for almost six weeks. After the ordeal of making my way through the hospital's systems, I went home and took a nap.

Our household goods arrived from Belgium in late July, and we spent the month of August unpacking and hanging wall paper. That probably helped my shoulder as much as anything. Late in the month, we took Sarah to Pennsylvania to start her freshman year at Lafayette College. It had been wonderful to have her with us in Texas for a month after being separated for so long.

I planned to return to work in September, and I sent my disability form to Provident informing them of that decision. To my surprise, a Provident agent called to ask about our relocation to Texas and about my current treatment.

"I think you should remain on disability for another month," she advised.

"Doesn't our policy state that I may not work at all if I'm on disability?" I asked. "I have a trip back to the company headquarters planned in September, so I'm probably required to end my disability payments."

"I think we can let you do that," she said. "In our experience, cancer patients who've had chemotherapy go back to work too soon. If you decide you need more time to recover after you have gone back to work, it will take you another three months without working to file for disability again. Why don't you stay on disability another month and see how you feel when you go to the office in September?"

In September, I attended an alumni leadership conference in Williamsburg and visited VIMA. I found it both energizing and tiring to get back into the swing of things. I returned to Texas sore and exhausted. I had spent a lot of time on my feet during very long days. The agent from Provident had been right.

Within my first two months in Texas, I managed to see all the specialists I needed except the surgeon. I spoke with the plastic surgeon about doing scar revision in the area where the drains had been under my arm. He patiently explained to me all the options for reconstruction, showed me photos, checked my stomach, and said I was a great candidate for a tummy tuck and TRAM flap; but again, I said no, thank you. Had I wanted reconstruction, however, I could not have had it until the physical therapy was finished and I had complete range of motion back in my arm.

The wig bothered me in the heat. Around the house, I went wigless with about an inch of hair. When I took Ashley for a hair appointment, I asked the hairdresser, "Do you think I have enough hair that you can highlight it?"

I removed the wig and she fingered my short hair.

"Sure," she responded, "we can highlight it and shape it."

On September 13, I sent out the news flash.

> *Dear friends,*
> *Since you have given me so much support in the last nine months,*
> *I wanted to share with you a great step forward. On Thursday, I*

had my one inch of hair highlighted, trimmed, and I "came out" at
a Chamber of Commerce dinner for 500 people. I'm not sure I feel
as though hair this short is the real "me," but it is a lot easier, more
comfortable and COOLER than the wig. I wore the wig or hats or
scarves for six months, so I feel like I've been freed.

My upbeat message did not reflect my absolute fear of going public with no more than one inch of hair. When I entered the Chamber of Commerce dinner, I felt the same insecurity I had felt at the party we attended the day after I received the diagnosis. I did not want Bob to leave my side. We sought out the few folks from Fort Hood whom we knew, and the wives were great at complimenting my new "do." We sat at a table with no one we knew, but by the end of the evening, I connected with Bob's dinner partner, also a breast cancer survivor. Members of our club were truly a magnet for one another.

Four days after I came out of the wig, I celebrated my forty-ninth birthday. I washed my hair that day and decided I had made a huge mistake. I could not do anything with my short hair. Psychologically, I did not want to go back into the wig after washing it and putting it away. But my short hair simply stood straight up and looked like a punk hairdo. I felt miserable. My only choice was to go out looking like a punk rocker or to wash my hair again and smooth it straight onto my head. I went out with my spike hairdo, feeling terribly self-conscious.

The next day, our neighborhood gathered together to surprise a friend on her fiftieth birthday. I felt sorry for myself. I strapped on the newly acquired TENS unit, slicked my hair down to my head, and Bob and I joined the surprise. My mood was as low as it had been in May as I came out of the chemo fog. I looked bad, my shoulder ached, and I felt more sick than optimistic that day.

A Bump in the Road

For four months, I had progressed steadily, gaining strength and energy, feeling my body healing. Suddenly, I hit a bump in the road. I recalled a letter from my childhood friend, Ruth.

Dear Barbara:

The main reason I wanted to write was to share my experience in terms of emotional recovery. I approached the actual surgery and the physical recovery period in a very matter-of-fact way. I knew what I had to do and I did it. In a way, it was like getting down to business. Emotions needed to be controlled, even postponed. The hospital informed me about the existence of support groups. But I didn't have any desire to belong to one. I thought I was handling things just fine.

The doubts and fears came later. Maybe nine months later. It wasn't rational (by definition). Rather suddenly, I was just afraid of death. Not the process of dying really, just death itself. What was odder still, the fear was not about what they had found. It was whether I had developed, and they had missed, something in a completely different place. After all, if I could develop cancer in one place, why not another? After letting that fear fester inside myself for longer than I should have, I spoke to my regular doctor. I think she listened to both what I said and how I said it. She told me that the evidence is incontrovertible. Health and recovery depends a lot on the emotional state. To put it in my own words, I was harming my physical health by not dealing with an emotional problem. She

141

advised me to talk to a professional, which I didn't. But I did work on it. I "talked" to myself, read some things, and then talked with some friends and advisors. That seemed to get me over the worst of it. I'm fully able to embrace life again and plan for the future rather than worry about the past. I suppose there will always be doubts but I'm not dwelling on them and they don't have a grip on me anymore.

I know that things occur differently for different people and I'm not suggesting that your experience will be or should be like mine. But I wanted to give you a "heads up" about something that caught me by surprise. In the period prior to the surgery and during the physical recovery I had a lot of caring, supportive people checking on me. But I continued to seem okay to them. After I was back in my day-to-day routine, that support faded into the background. It would have been there if I had asked for it, but it wasn't volunteered up.

So I guess what I'm saying is the following:

- *Don't be surprised if there's a rebound effect. I was absolutely blindsided by it and so I had to deal with that as well as the actual effect.*
- *It might help if you ask people to continue to be forthcoming about their support for some time after it doesn't seem necessary.*

My fears were not the same as Ruth's, but I clearly had an after-the-fact emotional response, and I found her experience helpful to consider. I did not know of anyone I could talk to. Being new, I did not know a personal or a professional resource. And the effort to get the attention of the medical community drained me.

I realized that the disability insurance folks were right. I had real limitations on my stamina while trying to balance an increased focus on work, playing general's wife, keeping up with about four or more medical appointments a week, and finishing the move into our new home.

The frequent medical appointments each week wore me down. Under the Army's new managed care system, I was limited in the amount of physical therapy allowed. To continue the physical therapy I needed, I must continually return to my primary care provider. Sometimes it took as many as four visits to get the proper paperwork to walk between the three buildings. The contractor balked at extending my care beyond eight weeks, yet my prognosis stated that it would take a year or more of continuous physical therapy to overcome the frozen shoulder. The internist sent me to an orthopedic surgeon to confirm the diagnosis. I explained to my mother:

October 9, 1997

> *I saw the orthopedic surgeon today. He looked at my x-rays from Belgium and said he wouldn't rule out surgery. But, he wants me to continue physical therapy. I've just gotten a phone call authorizing more physical therapy through November 14, but the paperwork hassle to get extensions on care is ridiculous. I had to go to three offices today to try to get an extension on my care. I was almost in tears by the time I got to the final lady who was able to work it out. But next time I ask for an extension, the approval has to go all the way to San Antonio to a civilian contractor who makes a profit on what he doesn't spend for health care. This is not good medicine.*

I wanted to get on with life, but it seemed as though life revolved around medical appointments and all of them required a fight. I knew that every time I walked into the managed care office with another request, they cringed. I was unwilling to accept a bureaucratic response counterproductive to good healing. And, I did not have the stamina nor the health to deal very well with the stress of repeatedly having roadblocks put in the way of recovery. I often reacted emotionally, explaining that the bureaucracy impeded my healing. They looked at me as a frozen shoulder, not as a cancer patient with physical and psychological needs.

On October 16, I met with the hospital commander.

"Do you know what it takes for a cancer patient to find the appropriate care in your hospital?" I asked him.

My voice shook and tears were very close as I talked to him. I did not appear as the professional chief executive officer, but rather as an emotionally fragile cancer patient.

The commander expressed his embarrassment that a cancer patient would have to fight the system so hard. He asked my help in improving the system. At the moment, though, I needed all my energy to focus on my own healing before I could take on the system for others.

In some ways, I felt as though I were leading a double life. I certainly functioned, going to social events, community meetings, and traveling. To my new friends who had not known me before nor seen me throughout the treatments, I appeared to be back to normal.

However, my mental state did not feel normal and the side effects of the tamoxifen, which I had begun taking in May following the chemotherapy, took their toll. My hot flashes increased and I had probably gained at least fifteen pounds, maybe more. We did not dress up a lot in Texas, but when we did, I found it increasingly difficult to find skirts, slacks and dresses I could wear. I finally decided to clear the closets of all the things that were too tight rather than look at clothes that did not fit. I packed up six large plastic leaf bags full of wonderful business suits, formals, and good clothes and took them to the thrift shop. I wrote to Kennon:

> *October 17, 1997*
>
> *I've felt terrible all week. I guess the emotional roller coaster goes with the whole ordeal. I see the surgeon for the first time on Monday and I get a mammogram tomorrow. I've started water aerobics and that is fun and energizing. Maybe it will help me combat the weight gain from the tamoxifen. We're going to Ashley's football game tonight and to a formal tomorrow night. Yesterday I tried on dozens of formals and cocktail dresses that I've been carrying around for years. I'm getting rid of all of them that don't look ravishing. No sense in thinking I'll lose weight and be able to wear them again.*

I went to physical therapy two days a week, and while my range of motion increased, I still had shoulder pain and incomplete movement. I received the same treatment I had in Belgium—electrical stimulation, range of motion and ice massage. Then, I performed overhead lifts on a machine with resistance, followed by pulling on an over-the-door pulley without resistance. At home, I did rotator cuff strengthening with a small dumbbell.

The water aerobics classes were enjoyable and seemed to help my shoulder as much as toning up the rest of my body. I felt awkward, however, when I went into the locker room to change. Most of the women did not mind changing in front of one another, but I always went into a stall so no one would see my mastectomy incision and flat chest. Actually, one of my more depressing moments had been the first time I put on a bathing suit. Bob told me that the special swim form was clearly the wrong size and he could tell the difference. After that, I always felt self-conscious.

In October, I had my first mammogram since the one that revealed the cancer. As I had been told I would, I felt some anxiety. Waiting for several days for the radiologist to read it brought back unpleasant memories and uncertainty, but it came back clean.

We ended the month on a high, Bob's fiftieth birthday on October 31. I surprised him with visits by Jenn, Sarah, his mother, and his aunt, and pulled off a small surprise party at home after Ashley's football game. For months I had worked on a secret gift for him that required the help of several friends more knowledgeable than I. We arranged a surprise delivery. With Bob busy entertaining his guests, the doorbell rang, and I encouraged him to answer the door. Upon opening it, he found the biggest surprise of all parked just outside: a 1977 white classic Corvette in near-mint condition, certainly able to drive over bumps in the road.

Thanksgiving

November brings Thanksgiving, arguably my very favorite holiday. The extended family planned to meet in Maryland at my mother's home, the same home where we had grown up as children. Kennon and Howard would be there, and it would give us all a chance to be grateful that the year of cancer had passed. My professional efforts had increased, and I began to feel more energy for work.

I had traveled to New York and to Chicago, making a presentation for my professional association. Scheduled to present at 3 p.m., I made a conscious effort during the day-long event to conserve energy so I could be "on" in the afternoon, my usual nap time.

Medical care continued. The quarterly oncology visit revealed low counts for both red and white cells, so I had not completely rebounded from the effects of chemo. The plastic surgeon revised the scar under my arm, and Dr. Day became my new hero. Although I did not succumb to his invitation for reconstruction, he was clearly a skilled surgeon. He completed the procedure in twenty-five minutes, and I was out of the hospital in an hour, with internal dissolvable stitches and steri-strips holding the skin together on the outside. I could even take a shower if I wanted. In physical therapy, I had reached about 90 percent range of motion and the pain in my shoulder had subsided. And, I now sported two inches of hair.

Just before Thanksgiving, Paddy wrote from Brussels:

November 24, 1997

Dear Barbara,
*   How many times I have composed letters to you in my head.*

146

Now, at this special time of year, I want to be sure I don't just depend on mental telepathy.

My first mental letters to you were composed during our nice beach vacation at Topsail, N.C. The weather was nice so every day I jogged up and down the streets, often passing a wonderful little tiny bookstore, and finally succumbing to its charms. Within I found a fine welcome. First, there was a great book called Warrior Women, *the title of which comes from the translation of the term "Amazon," women who fought to extraordinary lengths for their causes. It contains big photos of about twenty-five women who have had breast cancer, with about 100 words about each woman's journey. Excellent photography and text. I wanted the book, but it cost $50. So...after jogging around a bit more, I walked right in, introduced myself, told a little about our group, and asked if the owner would give it to us. As so often happens, this led to a nice conversation and mini-support group with the owner and her assistant. They each had friends who were in distress. Not only did she give me the book, she insisted I take another called* Recovering From Breast Surgery; Exercises to Strengthen Your Body and Relieve Pain, *by Diana Strumm, P.T. I love this woman to woman thing. It's so strong.*

I think all our ladies liked the books. I like to think of you and these women when I find life sometimes petty and jealous. It helps to reconfirm what's important.

That was a good reminder. We had traveled a lot of ground in the last year, and it was important to reconfirm what was important. On Thanksgiving day, I wrote to my e-mail support group:

Dear friends and family,

During the last eleven months, you have all been a tremendous support to me and have helped my healing through your prayers, your correspondence, your thoughtful phone calls and gifts, and frequent e-mail messages of love. I am thankful for each and every one of you.

Happy Thanksgiving.

Love,
Barbara

This message prompted a request from Willie in South Africa to explain Thanksgiving. He had seen pictures of families around the dinner table eating turkey, but he did not understand the tradition. It was a good exercise for me to think about the meaning for myself, and it reminded me of the Thanksgiving exactly one year before, the Thanksgiving b.c. (before cancer). We had been sad because Jenn and Sarah were not with us, so we hosted an international Thanksgiving, inviting NATO friends from Britain, Denmark, Belgium, Spain, France, and the U.S. As we sat down to dinner, Ashley explained the tradition of Thanksgiving, we all prayed together, and each person stated one thing for which he or she was thankful. That international Thanksgiving turned into the best one we ever had.

I explained to Willie:

The history of Thanksgiving is that in the early days of the colonies, the settlers from England had a very difficult time adapting to the new land, difficult weather, and very different natural foodstuffs. The first winter was very hard and many people died. Over the summer, the American Indians showed them how to use the native foods, how to work the soil, and how to plant and harvest in the new land. At harvest time, the colonials and the Indians sat down together to celebrate the successful harvest and their friendship. They gave thanks to God that they had enough food to last for the coming winter. It is interesting that Thanksgiving is a national holiday and a religious holiday, even though we have very firm separation of church and state. It is a family time, and is as important or more so than Christmas for families to get together.

It is always the fourth Thursday in November. The Wednesday before and the Sunday after are the most heavily traveled days of the year. Bob and I and our three daughters had a rendezvous at my mother's home in Maryland. My sister and her family came from Chicago. My stepsister and her family came from Philadelphia. There were fourteen of us living together for four days in my mother's house, and it was a wonderful reunion. My brother-in-law had been treated for colon cancer at the same time I was being treated for breast cancer, so it was a poignant reunion and we had much to be thankful for. I wish you could celebrate Thanksgiving with us someday.

Our weekend together in Havre de Grace was a wonderful celebration and reunion. As we took our turns around the dinner table telling what we were thankful for, there were some choked responses and teary eyes. Howard and I both celebrated putting a difficult year behind us. Together, we watched a television program describing several women's search for why breast cancer was becoming epidemic. But we could not stay serious for too long. As often happens when grown siblings get together, there is lots of reminiscence and fun. And we had to laugh at ourselves when the fourteen of us living in the house managed to stop up all the plumbing. Mother said she wanted us to remember the fun of being together, but we knew we would remember the plumbing problems first.

As a friend wrote from Belgium:

> *Life is so precious and being alive together with family and friends is one of the richest experiences we have. Happy Thanksgiving.*

'Tis the Season

After Thanksgiving, the days and weeks passing by felt rich and emotional with memories of the same time last year. I do not believe even my family understood how I relived each day of my cancer journey during this anniversary time. There were times when I was struck with what I had been doing on just this date last year. I would take a deep breath and close my eyes, sometimes holding back tears, and always being thankful that we were a year beyond the worst of the trauma.

We mailed our Christmas greetings early, sending our new address in Texas. I wanted people who only heard from us once a year to know that we had lived through a significant emotional event.

I kept the anniversary of December 10, the day of the fateful mammogram, to myself, as I had kept the news to myself the year before. Bob was traveling, as he had been the year before, and I shared with Ashley memories of that evening. There had been a Christmas "drinks party," as the Brits call cocktail parties, given by Bob's boss. I did not want to go when the time came, and the dread of the biopsy report must have put me in a pretty bad mood at home. Ashley had been glad to get rid of me and told me to stay a long time so she could have the house to herself. As the two of us ate dinner together a year later, I reminded her of that event and we laughed about our bad moods.

This year when Bob returned from his travel, I reminded him that it was just a year since he had taken me for the second biopsy. He acknowledged that, but did not want to relive each moment. So, with each passing day, I thought to myself, "This is what I was doing last year." Some of the memories were mere snippets.

I remembered the gentleness of the Belgian medical technicians during the second tissue biopsy. It took a long time and was quite uncomfortable, and they were very kind. I remembered the phone call from Chris Georgantopoulos and then my call to Bob, saying, "It's about as bad as it could be." I remembered our twenty-seventh wedding anniversary, wanting desperately to tell Bob that I had always dreamed of being married to him for fifty years and being unable to utter the words because of my tremendous fear. I remembered keeping the news to ourselves throughout the holiday season and Ashley's birthday celebration.

This Christmas would be far different than our sad, small Christmas the year before. All three girls would be home. Mother and my stepfather, Ed, joined us. We made a quick trip to San Antonio and had a delightful evening on the River Walk. We did not talk a lot about what we had been doing the year before at Christmas, but I felt very strongly that we were passing a significant marker, the year of cancer. I approached 1998 not only as a new year, but a year offering new promise and new beginnings. I knew that I was not quite the same person I had been. To others, I might appear to be the same Barbara, mother, daughter, sister, friend, but the last year had changed me forever.

Our friend Andy sent Christmas greetings about his cancer, and I was pleased that he mentioned me.

December 1997

The year started with our good friend Barbara Glacel informing us that she had cancer and was beginning treatment. The openness with which she was communicating with her friends (through e-mail, as she was in Belgium) was truly inspirational. It also proved to be supportive and helpful when Andy was diagnosed with prostate cancer. It made it much easier to immediately start talking about what to do. Fortunately Barbara said that she is about 90% improved and Andy is also doing well with the last test showing the PSA level "undetectable."

Christmas greetings brought shocked responses from folks who only heard from us once a year, and I found myself telling the story over and over. One friend sent an inspirational story that brought tears to my eyes.

December 22, 1997

Barbara,

I had no idea you have been so ill over the last year so I read your Christmas card with great interest. I have quite a bit of experience with cancer and chemo. My dad passed away in November 1978, my plebe year at West Point, following three years of chemo. Ironically, just as we received your card, my daughter, who obviously never knew my dad completed a short biography of him for her third grade class. You see, they had to write six short biographies on famous people, and after George Washington, Hans Christian Andersen and others, she asked if my dad was famous. Of course, as far as I am concerned he was, so Allie wrote a few paragraphs about him. I'll have to send it to you.

My dad was a carpenter and struggled to keep the family spoiled. When he got sick in 1975, he was at first misdiagnosed, but later it was clear he had cancer (mesothelioma) from asbestos inhalation at work. My uncle had my dad transferred from Peekskill to Boston to the Sydney Farber Cancer Center where he was treated, as well as at the Harvard Medical Hospital and Children's Hospital of Boston. At that time, chemo was in its infancy so everything they tried was experimental and voluntary. But my dad courageously tried everything and suffered the very uncomfortable side effects. About every six months the side effects would outweigh the benefits, and they would have to switch to another experimental drug. Eventually, they ran out of drugs they hadn't tried and he passed away. But thanks to my uncle's love, my dad's courage, and my mother's escorting him from New York to Boston every three weeks, we had him for another three years, and Sydney Farber learned a lot about chemotherapy. How exciting to learn that someone as wonderful as yourself was able to benefit from that, however indirectly. Thanks for keeping in touch, and have a Merry Christmas.

After Christmas, we traveled to Utah for our annual ski trip. The week on top of the mountain provided a time of healing and catharsis. I continued to keep the anniversary dates mostly to myself. I spent snowy mornings writing about the cancer experience, and sunny afternoons skiing down the slopes with my family. Taking a few black diamond runs was as much thrill as I wanted for 1998.

Part Four
Life

The world is round

and the place which may

seem like the end,

May also be only the

beginning.

—*Ivy Baker Priest*

Lifesavers

For my own mental health, I needed to put a period at the end of this sentence of my life. The move to Texas at the end of my chemotherapy treatment left me feeling incomplete about the chapter that took place in Belgium. Psychologically, at least for me, there was a real rite of passage to traverse at the anniversary of any trauma, and this was no exception. It had profound significance for me. On January 21, one year from the date of my second surgery at Jules Bordet, I spent some quiet time remembering and writing to those people who were my lifesavers at that most important time of my life.

Angela Shields, a nurse in the allergy clinic, had introduced me to Dr. Chris Georgantopoulos. Both of them were responsible for saving my life.

January 21, 1998

Dear Chris,

It was a year ago today that I had my second surgery. This last month has been full of memories of just what we were going through exactly one year ago. On December 30, I vividly recalled your going with Bob and me to Jules Bordet for the first time. It was terribly cold, we got very lost, and we slipped on the ice as we tried to maneuver our way across the sidewalk and street into the hospital. I was so grateful for your excellent French that got us through the reception process. Remember as we drove home, we saw where the tractor trailer had fallen off the overpass? They never fixed that guard rail before we left in July. I checked it out every time we drove by and remembered the events of December 30.

155

In many ways, things are back to "normal" now. But there is a new sort of normalcy. My new normal is a much less compulsive person. I find myself spending more time just sitting and enjoying, doing more reading, and also some writing rather than having to get work done.

I'm hoping that you and your family are settled back in Canada and happy to be home. Also hoping that your medical practice is appreciated for its value and high standards of care. I will forever be grateful that I met Chris Georgantopoulos at a time when I needed him. Thank you for all you've done for all of us.

January 21, 1998

Dear Madame Carstairs:

It was exactly one year ago this week that you visited me in the Jules Bordet hospital and talked to me about life after mastectomy. The thought of your visit and your kindness still brings tears to my eyes. Feeling somewhat lost as an American in the Belgian system, I had not expected to receive the advice that you had to offer. I will forever be indebted to you for reaching out to me.

Now that a year has passed since my treatment, I am able to join the Reach to Recovery program in the United States. I will go through the next training session, and I look forward to visiting other breast cancer patients. I would like to give to them what you gave to me, and it will help my own healing, I am sure. Whenever I visit a patient, I will think of you. Thank you from the bottom of my heart.

January 21, 1998

Dear Dr. Hertens:

It was one year ago that you and I went through a journey together at the Jules Bordet Clinic. During these past weeks, I have thought often of just what was happening one year ago. My first visit with you was on December 30, 1996, when Dr. Georgantopoulos, my husband and I traveled from Mons to consult with you. You immediately impressed us with your professional manner as well as your honesty and care for the patient. I felt very confident to be in your good hands, even with the terrible news that I had breast cancer. Throughout, I felt your support, I appreciated your advice, and I was grateful that you accepted my decisions even if they were not your first choice for treatment. Because you performed my surgery, I feel a special bond with you, and I am sorry I can not return to your clinic for follow-up.

I think of you often. I want you to know that I am very grateful to have met you one year ago. Thank you for your excellent care and kindness. I hope we will meet again some day.

Another crucial lifesaver in Belgium had been Marie Joris, my physical therapist. Marie worked with me for six months to reduce scar tissue, increase lymph drainage, and regain use of my shoulder and arm. Not only did her healing touch assist my recovery, but her willingness to help me work through the Belgian medical system was invaluable. I credit her, too, with providing me the treatment that gave me total feeling on my surgical site and no instances of lymphedema.

Dr. Jim Hines of Chicago had died several months earlier, so I wrote to his wife, Hollis.

January 21, 1998

When Kennon told me of Jim's death, I felt as though I had also lost a friend and supporter. It was exactly one year ago that I had surgery for breast cancer and had to make decisions about adjuvant treatment. The most difficult decision concerned chemotherapy since the Belgians did not recommend it and the Americans did. It proved so extremely helpful for me talk to a person of Jim's stature, as both a friend and a professional.

I remember quite well your answering the phone and our brief exchange and the warmth I felt from you over those 5000 miles. Jim was kind, clear, and decisive, which was just what I needed to "arm" myself to fight with the Belgian oncologists. Although I only spoke to each of you that one time, I felt that you were a true part of my support group that was scattered around the United States and pretty meager in Belgium.

I am so sad that Jim lost his own health battle. Please accept my sympathy and all good wishes and prayers for yourself during this difficult time. I will always be grateful for the gift that Jim gave to me.

My lifesavers at Walter Reed were Dr. Dave Jaques, Dr. Lou Diehl, and Jane Shotkin, R.N. I wrote to Dr. Diehl about my scattered care and asked his advice for what kind of follow-on tests I should be receiving. He explained that every three to four months, I should see a doctor to review any symptoms I might be having and talk over any new developments in the field of breast cancer. I should have a physical exam and blood work as needed, as well as review the current status of tamoxifen and required follow-up, particularly in light of the clinical trials underway using tamoxifen.

In addition, every twelve months I should have a mammogram and a gynecological evaluation by a gynecologist familiar with tamoxifen. Dr. Diehl invited me to come to Walter Reed for an appointment, and I decided that was a good idea. Shortly before I had my appointment with him, Kennon called with the disturbing news that there were dark areas in her latest mammogram and she had been called back for an ultrasound. She would have to wait for two weeks for the next appointment. Even knowing that most questionable mammograms turn out to be false alarms, I could not think of anything encouraging to say given my own history. Her two-week wait was agony for all of us, and I was ready to take the next plane to Chicago on the day she had the ultrasound.

My visit with Dr. Diehl was both reassuring and a little unsettling. In his patient manner, he answered every question thoroughly. He later told Jane Shotkin that I was "starved for real information." He even talked to me about Kennon's mammogram, saying that in a woman's fifties, often the dark areas on mammograms are simply the breast tissue beginning to break down. Later, when I wrote to him to say that was exactly her diagnosis, he responded, "The day I go out of business will be a great day...I am delighted that your sister's mammogram and ultrasound did not demonstrate a more serious problem."

The unsettling part of the conversation concerned the practice of not performing routine screening tests such as bone scans or liver scans. I knew that in Belgium, I would have all those tests at the one-year mark. Dr. Diehl explained that it is not common practice in this country. Rather, a cancer patient must be attuned to symptoms—for instance, headaches, a persistent cough, aches in joints and bones, or irregular blood counts. Any of these symptoms might indicate a metastasis and should be investigated immediately. Suddenly I knew why cancer survivors often felt like hypochondriacs.

Before leaving the hospital, I visited Jane Shotkin, the helpful oncology nurse, and Dr. Dave Jaques, the surgeon who had been my lifeline when I first received diagnosis. I learned then that he was going to Memorial Sloan Kettering, and I pledged to follow him if I ever needed more surgery.

At the next visit to my internist back in Texas, I explained to her what Dr. Diehl had said about symptoms, and then I reeled off every ache and pain I had. She did not think I was being an alarmist. Her own mother had died at age forty of breast cancer, and she lives in fear that she will have cancer. She immediately booked me for a chest x-ray, x-rays of my elbows which were aching, blood work, a vaginal and uterine ultrasound, and a consult to the chief of gynecology. She also offered to see my three daughters to talk to them about breast self-exams and early detection.

Over the next several months, I became a regular in the gynecology department. Tamoxifen has the unfortunate side effect of increasing the risk for endometrial cancer of the uterus. I had a small amount of spotting, but even that was enough for concern. When the doctor suggested a uterine biopsy, my experience of twenty-five years earlier came immediately to mind, and I asked if they had perfected the technique at all. Again, the doctor said it would not be very painful. Again, I wondered how a man without a uterus could ever say that. Yet, the procedures were intended to save my life and were therefore welcomed.

In May 1998, the physical therapy finally ended with full range of motion back in my arm. It seemed strange to have a full day available to me and not be going to see the physical therapists who had become friends by now. Peno Carter and Linda Pace had stretched me back to normal over a period of nine months, a symbolic time for giving new life.

I am grateful to the lifesavers who saw me through the surgery and chemotherapy, and to those who now continue to "hold" me, in the words of Jim Hines, through my new life as a cancer survivor. They are an important part of my life insurance and longevity.

Role Models

When we first returned to the United States, we spent a few days at my childhood home with my mother. There is always such a feeling of comfort in going home. After the trauma of the previous six months, being in my childhood home felt wonderful. My mother had always been a role model for me. A successful businesswoman, she endured several tragedies as a young mother and she always survived with grace. When my father died, she was only forty-one years old. She took over the family business and rose to national prominence in her industry. The thoughts of her strength and positive attitude had led me through my own crisis, and I strived to meet her ideal.

Another role model was my mother's friend Bea, the first person I had ever known to have breast cancer. She visited me at Mother's. More importantly, she had helped me through my treatment via mail and e-mail. I had been in college when Bea was diagnosed with breast cancer. I remembered her coming to the house during the time of her radiation treatments. I could see the markings on her skin to direct the radiation. I knew that she had a radical mastectomy at that time, and I was astounded when she described to me the details after my own surgery.

Dear Barbara,

I am a volunteer with Reach to Recovery, an arm of the American Cancer Society, and therefore I call on breast cancer patients. You may remember that I had a radical mastectomy almost thirty years ago, on March 9, 1967. I tell you this because I hope it will give you encouragement. I was forty-four years old at the time. Medical treat-

*ment has changed and advanced a lot since then. There were no
mammograms or chemotherapy then; and the radical procedure is
not done today. My prognosis was very poor; nine of the ten lymph
nodes removed were positive for medullary cancer. According to statistics at the time, I had one year to live. Thank goodness, I was not
told this until many years later. Only when I learned of my prognosis
did I fully understand my husband's reaction. My treatment consisted of five daily injections of theratepa and five weeks of radiation.
I know I am lucky and thank the good Lord every day. I hope you
have a positive attitude because I am convinced that helps so much. I
know many women who have had the same good luck that I have
had and pray that you, too, will receive the same providence.*

I was astounded as I thought of that prognosis of thirty years before.
Bea had continued to live a full and active life, worked in her husband's
surgical clinic, was an active community volunteer and a grandmother. In
fact, she had outlived her husband. Her example gave me tremendous
hope. When she learned of my diagnosis, she sent materials from the
American Cancer Society. I responded to her:

*I have been thinking of you since long before I received your
package, and wanting to write to you since then. Somehow, I don't
have much energy for sitting down to write, but I'm keeping up
with folks quite well through e-mail.*

*First, thank you for all the wonderful information you sent and
the inspirational letter as well. You are not being intrusive at all—
just caring and loving, and I appreciate it so much.*

*You don't realize that I have been thinking of you since Decem-
ber 20 when I got the confirmation that I had breast cancer. You
are the first person I ever knew who had it, and you are such a role
model. I remember clearly the summer you were having radiation
treatments. You were so positive then and your grace in dealing
with the effects for all these years has been tremendous. I kept saying
to Bob that you had survived and I could too. That is not to say that
there haven't been down times and lots of fears, but the optimistic
times are more often. I can't adequately express to you how much I
have felt you with me for the last two months. Thank you.*

Lynne wrote to me about the wife of a mutual friend who also served as a role model when I was down. She said:

> *Jack has been wanting to send you a note but it's been hard. Their children were still in grade school when his wife was first diagnosed with breast cancer which had already spread throughout her body. Her first prayers were to see the girls graduate from high school, then college, then married, then to see the grandchildren. Her strength kept her going over twenty-five years, until last year. She was able to baby-sit five of their six grandchildren.*

I identified with these thoughts as I vividly remembered my emotions at the time I was diagnosed. I fervently wanted to live long enough to see my girls be happy, get married, have children. At that time, I had seen two of them graduate from high school, but there were so many life events ahead that I wanted to share with them.

When I thought of these courageous ladies, I knew there was hope for me. Even when I was in the worst state emotionally, I could call up the images of these survivors. I also thought of my friend Marilyn. Marilyn had multiple sclerosis and bravely battled the disease as it began to take away her ability to walk and sometimes slurred her speech. She would not let it get her down. She continued to swim and ride horses in order to painfully exercise the muscles that did not want to work any more. I felt that I must follow Marilyn's example in my own illness. I told Lynne:

> *When I feel down, I think about two people who are such an inspiration to me: Max and Marilyn. Then I realize that I don't have anything to complain about, and I can get on with life.*

Max had died of leukemia just one year before I was diagnosed with cancer, and he was another very strong role model to me. The treatments he received brought him close to death on more than one occasion. He allowed the doctors at Johns Hopkins, at Walter Reed, and at Brooke Army Medical Center to experiment on him with every kind of drug and treatment possible. He was the third human ever to receive the GCSF treatment to stimulate recovery of the bone marrow. He was one of the very first to harvest his own bone marrow for subsequent transplant. He was the friend for whom Ashley had drawn the purple amoeba to remind him that the deadly poisons in the chemotherapy were his friends. Often when I was fighting with the Belgian doctors to allow me to receive chemotherapy in Belgium, I thought of Max. It was also his lead that I followed in consciously choosing my photos and symbols for my hospital visits.

My friend John served as a role model too. Throughout several years of surgery and chemotherapy for lung cancer, John never lost his work ethic, his drive for perfection, his caring about other people, and his will to live. He worked as the Athletic Director at William and Mary up until just days before he died. He was known for leaving meetings to receive chemotherapy injections and coming straight back before the meeting ended. He looked at the positive side of life, and he gave spirit to other cancer patients through the local support group. John had lost his battle on the very day we had moved to Belgium, and I remember flying overnight and crying on the plane. But his life spirit was an inspiration and a statement of hope.

When I felt the most upset and depressed, these role models gave me hope. It helped me to think I might provide this kind of example to others. Many friends gave me the encouragement to have hope and continue the fight. From my Finnish daughter, Keiju, I also had hope for the future.

Dear Mom,

I hope you are feeling ok. I am more than sorry that I haven't written you earlier. It is somehow really hard for me to deal with the situation when someone I love is hurting because of an illness, for example. It is extremely hard for me to find the right words. But I want you to know that you are in my prayers, and I have a habit of thinking about the people who I really care about just before falling asleep as I lay in my bed and I do think of you every night. Mom, I know that you are such a determined person, and in fact a real fighter, that you won't give up, never, am I right?

I apologize for not writing you earlier. That does not mean that I don't care or that I have forgotten you. No. It is just that cancer is one of the things that I just don't understand. Every time I hear of cancer I ask myself why, why, why. Maybe that is one of the many reasons why I want to become a doctor. I want to be there for people when they need me and to be able to help them. So, I guess that's one of my goals in life and in being a doctor. For quite a long time now I have also wanted to become a researcher as well as a doctor, and try to find a cure for cancer.

> *Love you lots,*
> *Keiju*

The thought of Keiju finding a cure for cancer provided much hope. In 1998, she entered medical school in Turku, Finland, and was accepted into the prestigious research program.

Reach Out and Touch Someone

During my treatment, I had longed so for others to reach out and touch me that I became obsessed with reaching out to touch others. Every night as I lay in bed, I prayed by name for everyone I knew who had cancer. Often I had not even met these people, but they were friends of friends whose names I heard through my e-mail support group. The prayer list grew longer and longer, and continues to do so. There are now so many names that I may forget someone or sometimes even fall asleep before I finish the list. I vary the order of names so that if I fall asleep before finishing, I still pray by name for everyone several times a week. I pray for those undergoing treatment first; and then by geographic area, I pray for survivors, asking that they remain cancer-free.

While still in Belgium, during my first round of chemotherapy, I learned of a young American Army wife who had been diagnosed with cancer and would be receiving treatment at Jules Bordet with Dr. Hertens. Because the medical clinic did not support our support group, the doctors refused to give us the names of new patients and would not tell the new patients that we existed. I learned through Chris about this new patient, but he did not know her name. I also heard that the young woman was, understandably, very upset, and that the young female doctor treating her had never treated a breast cancer patient before. Sometimes these young and inexperienced doctors could be quite arrogant, perhaps in their own insecurity and inexperience. They felt threatened by a support group and feared we were dispensing medical information. They refused our invitations to attend our meetings to see how supportive and nonmedical we were.

Having learned a few things about Jules Bordet after my two weeks of residence, I wanted to pass on some information to this new patient about surviving in a Belgian hospital. I had been told that she was only twenty-nine years old and spoke not one word of French. I frantically tried to find her. Finally, the head nurse at the hospital agreed to give my note and two books to the new patient. I told her about the hospital routine, what to take with her, and how to ask for the *bessin de lit*. I encouraged her to read *Joining the Club* and *Dr. Susan Love's Breast Book* that accompanied the note. And I asked her to call me if I could help.

Dee did call me right away. I talked to her while she was in the hospital and we were able to share laughter about some of the hospital events and the terrible food. She joined our support group and kept us laughing even as she had terrible complications from her surgery and made frequent trips to Bordet. She followed up with both radiation and chemotherapy. One doctor had suggested to Dee that she see a psychiatrist because she was too happy. Dee's happiness came from her family and the Lord. She had a very strong faith, and her church community rallied around her. I left Belgium before Dee did, and during my last weeks there, I took meals to her and her family. It made me feel so good to give to someone else as Nancy had given to me, remembering that cancer treatment takes a long time and one continues to need the touch of friends for many months.

Just before leaving Belgium, I received a disheartening message from a business colleague and one of my e-mail support group.

June 30, 1997

Dear Barbara,

I'm afraid that I have some bad news to report, and that is that I have joined a not-so-exclusive club that you belong to...women who have breast cancer. I'm terrified, I'm encour-aged, I'm...well you probably know...I'm in a different world than I was a month ago.

Lots of love,
Shannon

I felt devastated by Shannon's message. She was way too young to have breast cancer. At thirty-eight, she had a three-year-old son and a busy ca-reer. She, too, had hit the wall. I immediately responded to her with all the information and advice I could put into a message. I tried to remember all the details of the last six months to ease her fear of the unknown. As she went through her treatment, we became frequent correspondents.

Providing hope to others is what the American Cancer Society Reach to Recovery program is all about. I thought often about the ray of hope that had walked into my hospital room on the day that Madame Carstairs arrived. I wanted to be that ray of hope to others. To become a Reach to Recovery volunteer, one must be one year beyond treatment with no complications of lymphedema or recurrence. While I had to wait until 1998 to be a volunteer, it did not stop me from trying to provide comfort to other breast cancer patients.

Having had cancer, one is drawn to other cancer patients like a magnet. Shortly after we arrived in Texas, I learned of a wife whose husband worked for Bob who was having cancer surgery. I called her before we even met formally. Faith had family in the area and was well supported, but we still had an immediate bond. She puts things in perspective when she says that after having cancer, when she stubs her big toe, she is convinced she has a metastasis and has cancer of the big toe. It sounds funny, but the feeling often isn't. Only another cancer patient understands that.

Within six weeks of our arrival, we learned about a young wife with cancer and a horror story of delays in receiving treatment. Her husband had been assigned to Korea and was brought home on a compassionate reassignment. He requested that his boss give him a flexible schedule so he could help care for Toni and their young son. When Bob received the request, he immediately brought it home to me, and he responded favorably to the request. I called Toni and then other wives in the command. We arranged for meals, emergency child care, and other needs for the family during the many months ahead while Toni had two major operations, two rounds of chemo, and then a stem cell transplant. Through this whole terrible ordeal, Toni was a trooper. She did not like her wig, so she went bald with bright lipstick and big earrings. She did not like the prosthesis, so she draped colorful scarves over her flat side. She answered the phone saying "Praise the Lord," and she was determined to survive despite grim medical findings. We reached out to touch her, but she touched the many people who met her. She would call me when she heard of other women having trouble receiving care, and we would join forces to make the system respond to them.

As soon as I reached a year from my treatment, I went through the American Cancer Society training to be a Reach to Recovery volunteer, and now I officially reach out to touch others as Madame Carstairs reached out to me. It provides hope to me as well as to others.

Warrior Women

Paddy had written about the book she got for the Belgian support group, *Warrior Women*, about the Amazon women known for their prowess in battle. I also thought of what Bridgette had told me a year before in Jules Bordet, about the Amazon women elite who cut off their right breasts in order to shoot the bow and arrow better. As I felt better, I was ready to assume that role. I had already lost my right breast, and I had a history of fighting for a cause.

On the same day that I saw Dr. Diehl, I stopped at the Pentagon to see the Deputy Assistant Secretary of Defense for Health Affairs. His request set the ball rolling for my fight for improved access to medical care for military families. His wife had had two frozen shoulders, and he understood that the treatment is both very painful and very long-term. He was appalled that the medical director in our region did not know that. He encouraged me to write down the problems I had experienced in getting care. In past months I had resisted writing about it, because I knew it would take a long time. By now, however, I had more stamina and the ability to focus on detail which I had lost during the chemo fog, so I undertook that monumental task. I wanted to improve the system so that seriously ill patients would not have to expend their limited energy in working through the bureaucracy to find the doctors who might hold them through treatment.

Not only did I have to frequently run the gamut of multiple appointments to get authorization for continued physical therapy, but the system started sending back paperwork for ridiculous reasons. One such snafu was set in action by the contractor who issued me a portable TENS unit for my shoulder after my arrival in Texas. Several months later, I received a letter stating I had not secured the proper permission and I must go to the issue office. No one seemed to know the location of the issue office, and I was directed from one building to another, then to the basement, then to the soiled linen department, then to the loading dock. Finally a kind person told me that the issue office had been eliminated and taken over by the contractor more than a year earlier—the same contractor who sent me on the wild goose chase.

The system's paperwork process was so poor that my physical therapist was not being paid, and I was not receiving receipts that would allow me to collect from my supplemental insurance policy. In March, I wrote to a friend:

> *I am convinced that the TRICARE system has a red flag on my file that says "Apply Murphy's Law to every action." Latest is that they kicked back my claim for payment for a prosthesis because mastectomy was written in the wrong box by the doctor and they had no diagnosis. Now really—can you think of any other reason someone would order an artificial boob?*

With every mistake they made, my documentation simply grew longer. I reached the end of my rope on a day when I again followed up on a request for extension of physical therapy treatment. The nursing supervisor had promised to call me several days earlier with the response to my request, but I had received no phone call. When I mentioned that, she yelled at me that I was lying and said she had better things to do than to call patients. The warrior woman took over. I addressed a letter to the Assistant Secretary of Defense for Health Affairs and sent copies to members of Congress, lobbyists, and the military leadership.

> *March 9, 1998*
>
> *The purpose of this letter is to convey information to you about the shortcomings of the TRICARE system in meeting medical needs of service members and families. Last month, I met personally with your deputy about these concerns. He requested that I document my case and send it to you in writing.*
>
> *As I have put together my record of events for you, I am struck*

with the blandness of listing the dates and events on paper. The two-dimensional black and white description of my fifteen-month health care saga fails to convey my true sense of outrage that the medical system is apparently so unconcerned with my life. When I reach the doctors, I find concern and care. The journey to reach those doctors, however, is fraught with bureaucratic nonsense that sick people should not have to endure. If I, as the wife of a senior ranking officer, still suffer the hassles of the system and the some-times-incompetence of the administrators, just imagine what our young soldiers and their families, who lack the horsepower and experience to overcome the obstacles, are suffering.

I outlined my personal problems in accessing care, and I took the opportunity to write about Toni:

The even sadder story of Toni, the wife of a staff sergeant at Fort Hood, is one that must also be told. Toni discovered a lump in her breast in May 1997 while her husband was assigned to Korea. Toni made a same-day appointment and saw a doctor who ordered an immediate mammogram. Toni walked her paperwork to Radiology to make an appointment. The receptionist there told her that because she was thirty-two and had no history of breast cancer in her family, that she probably just had calcifications and did not need an immediate mammogram. The receptionist, ignoring the doctor's orders, booked an ultrasound for three weeks later. At the time of the ultrasound, the technician exclaimed, "Oh my God, that's huge." Nonetheless, she scheduled Toni for a routine mammogram another three weeks later. Following the mammogram, no one called Toni with results. Toni called the Family Care Clinic and found no one who would help her to locate the original doctor who had ordered the mammogram, nor anyone else who would get the results for her. Toni could feel the tumor growing. After nine weeks from the original appointment, Toni opted out of the Army hospital care and booked an appointment at the local civilian hospital. The civilian doctor requested her records and made the diagnosis of cancer. The tumor had grown from the size of a walnut to the size of a grapefruit.

In August 1997, Toni had a mastectomy followed by chemotherapy. Her husband returned from Korea on compassionate reassignment. By November, the cancer had returned and invaded the chest wall. In December, Toni had surgery to excise the chest wall, and she continued on chemotherapy. On March 8, Toni entered the Texas Cancer Institute in San Antonio for a stem cell transplant. Her prognosis is not good. Because the system failed her, Toni is paying cost-share fees to receive civilian care. Even those cost-share fees are a drain on a staff sergeant's salary, especially in the situation where Toni has lost her job and child care fees are increasing due to Toni's illness. Toni's cancer is very aggressive, and the nine weeks of delay caused in part by the cost-saving orientation of TRICARE may, in fact, cost her her life.

I am serving now on a process action team at the Army hospital to help improve the management of care provided to those who have serious, long-term health concerns, particularly when they arrive at this military hospital in the midst of their treatment. This effort for improvement is heartening. However, the system moves far too slowly to save some lives that are at risk today. As I listen to the discussion from representatives of managed care, TRICARE, the civilian contractor, and the hospital, I am often disheartened that the primary goal is cost savings over patient health. There are times when I must remind them that the patient is the raison d'être of the entire system. This contradiction in mission is at the root of the problem of the TRICARE contract and its operation.

Military families deserve better. We move around the world, suffer hardships and separations, offer our beloved military members to a career where the ultimate sacrifice is not unexceptional, and we deserve better care. Good health care for families is a readiness issue as well as a moral issue.

Bob had said in jest for years that he continued to get promoted in spite of me, not because of me. In reality, he backed every effort I made to improve the quality of life for military families. We knew this letter might rock the boat within the military medical chain of command, but in the regular Army, I was actively cheered on. Generals to privates were having trouble with TRICARE, and they were glad to have someone voice their concerns.

In April, the National Military Family Association invited me to testify before a congressional committee holding hearings about opening the federal civil service medical programs to military families. I would be allowed five minutes for an oral statement and could submit an accompanying written statement for the record. My diary of treatment and hassles over the previous nine months now totaled forty-five pages. As Congressman Mica recognized me, he said:

> *I am pleased to welcome to our panel our second witness, Dr. Barbara Glacel, and I highly recommend her full testimony. She won't be able to give that here today. In fact, I am not sure that we can afford to print it—it is so lengthy—in the record, but we should also send the leadership a copy of her full documentary of her unbelievable experience with military health care and TRICARE when we appeal for action on this legislation. I have never seen anything so well-documented, Dr. Glacel, and I compliment you and I recognize you now for your testimony.*

I had practiced the statement several times to ensure the five minutes length. However, I ad libbed a few comments and spoke a little more slowly. When I had one minute remaining, a warning light went on. As I continued to speak, I felt a little panicked about what I would do when the buzzer sounded before I finished. However, Mr. Mica leaned over and turned off the light, a clear indication that what I was saying was worthwhile and that I could finish.

> *Thank you, Mr. Chairman, Mr. Cummings. Thank you for giving me the opportunity to testify today. I am sorry that I have this story to tell you, but I am glad that you want to listen.*
>
> *My message is that the TRICARE medical system is an impediment to good health, and difficulty in access actually deters the achievement of quality medical care. My struggles to achieve access to care have left me with the impression that TRICARE administrators believe breast cancer is no more significant than the common cold.*
>
> *If an educated woman with twenty-eight years of experience with the military has difficulty understanding and satisfying the bureau-*

cratic requirements; if the wife of a senior ranking officer must fight to obtain access to care, then I shudder to think what the privates, sergeants, and lieutenants and their families are suffering under TRICARE. I know of several breast cancer patients who have had such difficulty in gaining access to TRICARE Prime that their cancers have progressed to more serious stages before they were provided treatment.

I was diagnosed with breast cancer in December 1996 while my husband was assigned in Belgium. In 1997, I had two major operations and three months of chemotherapy in Belgian hospitals. During this time, I received physical therapy three days a week for complications following surgery. During chemotherapy, I lost considerable range of motion in my shoulder. Three doctors advised it could be one to two years of continuous therapy to regain range of motion because the effects of the chemicals caused additional problems of bursitis, tendinitis, and intraarticular effusion.

In July 1997, my husband was transferred to Fort Hood, Texas, within TRICARE Region 6. As a cancer patient, my highest priority was to re-establish medical care. My forty-five pages of written testimony outline the difficulties of the last nine months as I have fought the system for access to care. A few examples must suffice in this brief testimony.

- *TRICARE promises that specialty care will be provided within twenty-eight days of a consult. My referral to orthopedic surgery took forty-seven days. Therefore, I walk through my own consultation paperwork which means going to three separate buildings in different locations, waiting three times, and in one location merely having an employee put a stamp on a piece of paper.*
- *The TRICARE contractor authorized purchase of a portable TENS unit for my shoulder. Four months later, I received a letter from the contractor telling me I had not supplied proper paperwork. The TRICARE representative sent me to the main hospital where I was directed through the basement, onto the loading dock, through soiled linens, and into the warehouse only to discover that the TRICARE contractor had taken over the function of this nonexistent office some nine months earlier.*

- *A total of six medical doctors confirmed that my condition required continuous long-term treatment, probably for over a year. Yet, every four to eight weeks, I am required to get more paperwork to be sent to an administrator 100 miles away to review whether I can continue care. During the last nine months, I have had care decreased from the prescribed three days a week to one day a week. I have had care discontinued or threatened discontinuation. I have had administrators tell me incorrect procedures for how to get authorization for more care. The system has taken more than the authorized time in reviewing my request in several instances; and I have even had a TRICARE nursing supervisor yell at me that I was lying and she had more important things to do than to call patients.*

- *The TRICARE system looks at me as a series of specific symptoms, not as a complex body in which breast cancer may affect my brain, lungs, liver, and bones. At the same time that the TRICARE administration was threatening to discontinue my physical therapy, three surgeons were telling me that I might need surgery to correct the shoulder problems, but I couldn't have surgery until physical therapy got me to an extended range of motion. This was the proverbial Catch 22. Do we save money in the short term by not giving me more physical therapy treatment? Only to spend a lot more later on surgery which will require even more physical therapy?*

As a cancer patient, I have both physical and psychological healing required for recovery. The TRICARE system directly impedes my healing. I simply do not have the stamina to cope with bureaucrats who are either incompetent or untrained, an administrative system that does not consider the prescription from the medical care provider, and a system with access that is so difficult that it is easier to ignore my own health concerns.

If someone with my experience and the rank of my husband to open doors cannot obtain access to medical care, I do not believe that the soldiers and their families who protect this country can either. It is a readiness and retention issue for our Armed Forces, as well as a moral issue to military members and families.

At the end of my oral statement, Mr. Mica confirmed by unanimous consent that my entire written testimony would be made part of the Congressional Record. After the other witnesses on our panel spoke, we responded to questions. Mr. Mica stated again that he was glad that he put my whole written statement in the record because it provided the documentation and detail for the first time showing how an individual struggled with the system just to receive access to care. He commented that it did not seem compassionate nor user-friendly. I agreed with him, noting that I had less difficulty working through the medical system in a foreign language than I had working through TRICARE.

Within a few days, I had hit the front page news in the syndicated Cox newspaper chain, our local *Killeen Daily Herald*, my hometown newspaper in Maryland, and inside pages in the *Navy Times* and the *Army Times*. The *Navy Times'* quote for the week was my statement: "The system itself impedes the very purpose for which the system was created." The local paper screamed, "General's Wife Fights TRICARE." A subsequent letter to the editor was headlined "Hail to TRICARE fighter." The *Army Times* headline said, "Caught in the System—Military wife must battle TRICARE and breast cancer."

The response was incredible. I don't know how people found me, but I received phone calls, e-mails, and letters from people around the country whom I did not know. One hundred percent of the responses were positive. Many people wanted me to listen to their horror stories and tell Congress. Some wanted to offer their help to me and solutions for healing my frozen shoulder. Others offered prayers and sympathy.

The three top executives of the contractor organization flew in from California to talk to me. They had reviewed all my paperwork, and incredibly, they found some billing errors that not even I had found. Nonetheless, even after another six months of trying to settle the paperwork hassles, there remained two invoices that they had sent incorrectly so many times that I stopped trying to correct the errors. I had spent more in time and money mailing papers back and forth than I could collect from my supplemental insurance.

The Surgeon General of the Army and his deputy both wrote to not only apologize, but to let me know that they had sent my testimony to every TRICARE region in the country, asking whether similar problems existed. They reported that new TRICARE contracts lifted the requirement for preauthorization for physical therapy.

Legislation passed as a result of the committee hearings, authorizing a test project for military retirees, but not for active duty families. My local hospital implemented a plan to better identify and track incoming chronic-care patients, a plan to which I contributed through membership on a process action team. However, problems with access to the system continued to plague seriously ill patients. Unfortunately, the hospital administration and the contractor that managed the care continued to state that these "unique" cases were not the norm for patient care under their system, and so they resisted further action to correct the systemic problem. It seems to me that every patient situation is unique, and that if the most seriously ill patients are too unique to get access, then I still question whether the system is not impeding progress toward its very mission. The National Military Family experts reported "...the way the current program is structured, it will never provide managed care. Your case is the typical one; the contracts do not require managed care and the system does not allow managed care."

I knew it would take more than one warrior woman to change this dinosaur.

What Goes Around Comes Around

Surviving the cancer battle is a team effort. My friend Jani had sent me a book, *Where the Buffaloes Roam*, describing the team that cancer patient Bob Stone put together to help him fight cancer. He described the buffalo as an animal that had become nearly extinct and had put up a valiant and successful fight to survive, thus he named his support team The Buffaloes. My team had begun with about twenty folks whom we e-mailed, wrote or called in the first days of my journey to recovery. When I sent out my last messages of thanksgiving for their support eleven months later, this team had grown to 100 just on e-mail, and many others who stayed in touch through telephone, letter, and personal visits.

Our friend Bea, one of my biggest supporters, introduced me to the American Cancer Society Relay for Life just as I finished my chemotherapy treatments. She and my mother lit candles for Howard and me that would burn throughout the duration of the relay as teams walked all night long to raise funds for cancer research. She wrote to me:

> *I lit a luminary in your honor. The luminary ceremony was very moving. There were about a thousand luminaries— more than could be placed around the track in a single line; a second line was started. As soon as it became dark, all lights on the field were extinguished and the luminaries were lighted. There were moving speeches and prayers and soft music. I was glad to be a part of it. I like to think of it as a celebration of life.*

Other friends wrote about participating in similar walks in Colorado,

New York, Washington, D.C. A colleague participated in the Revlon walk in Los Angeles and wrote:

> *Just a note to share a memento of the Revlon Run/Walk for Cancer and my nine-year-old daughter's journal entry from that day. I was thinking of you. It was all very inspiring.*

Her daughter wrote:

> *On Saturday, our family went to a Revlon walk for cancer. Forty thousand people came. They also had hats that people who survived wore. So my mom wore one because she had it and survived. I think that when you walk it shows that you care and that you're fighting not with your hands, but with your feelings. At the end of our three miles, we all ran through a tunnel that football players run through and we got a medal (brass). As we were walking, I saw my mom's eyes water because it was such a good feeling to have survived that terrible experience. I'm glad we went because it made my mom very happy.*

Bev had sent her pink survivor's hat to me, and that made me cry.

Rhonda had participated for several years in the Louisville Race for the Cure. I suggested to my college roommate, Lin, and Rhonda that the three of us could rendezvous in Louisville for the October 1998 race. A few weeks before the race, I participated in an American Cancer Society (ACS) effort to remind friends about doing breast self-exams and having annual mammograms. I sent 150 e-mail messages, informing of the ACS guidelines. I ended the message with a plea for financial sponsorship in the Louisville Race for the Cure.

I was astounded at the response to my message, and even now, it brings tears to my eyes. Within hours of sending the message, I got the first response from another sorority sister, sending contributions in honor of both Rhonda and me.

This was the first of many contributions for breast cancer education and research. When the first $100 check arrived from a business colleague, I literally wept. The generosity of the contributors was overwhelming. There were checks ranging from $25 to $500, and every one came with a note of love and encouragement. Bob didn't understand why I cried every time I opened another envelope. It was just wonderful.

The reunion weekend was full of good memories, poring over photo albums, talking about our college days together and all that had happened in the thirty years since we had first met. Each of us had experienced life-changing events. Rhonda had contracted both thyroid cancer and breast cancer. Lin's only child had died at two years of age from congenital defects. We all knew that one got through those hard times only because of the love and support of others.

On the day of the race, we joined 4500 others to race for the cure. Survivors had special hats and pink shirts. We all wore signs on our backs with names of survivors or victims of breast cancer. We posted white flags in a special area with the names of other survivors and victims. As Rhonda, Lin, and I walked together, we passed families with the names of mothers or sisters who had died, and I would get choked up as I read the names. The race was only three miles, but we who were survivors had run our marathons in our battle with cancer. This was a symbolic distance.

My family keeps up the effort for me year round. Always supportive and understanding, they pulled out the stops for my fiftieth birthday. Bob accepted the "Corvette Challenge" of eleven months before, and he pulled off the biggest surprise of my life.

I had planned to join Bob at the end of an Army trip to Australia. As I prepared for the trip, I found a note from Bob that read: "The trip is longer than you thought. Bring a nice dress for our last night." Curious, I looked through the airline tickets and discovered that after Australia, we were going to Bangkok and would actually be there on my birthday.

September fifteenth was the big day. We had breakfast in the suite and then spent the day shopping. After a sumptuous buffet lunch at the Oriental Hotel, we were driven to Johny's Gems. The employees, Johny, his wife, and his son expressed joy that we had returned to Bangkok. They served us drinks, and Bob explained that it was my birthday. They proceeded to show me the ugliest jewelry one could imagine. I tried so hard to be tactful, meanwhile thinking, "Oh my word, we came all this way for this tacky jewelry?"

Finally, and with a huge grin, Johny's son produced a large red box, saying, "I think we have something you'll like."

When he opened it, I was absolutely speechless. It had clearly been made especially for me. As Bob explained, I learned that for the past six months, he had been searching for a brooch. When he could not find one he liked, he designed one himself. He made a list of the important events in my life for the past fifty years. He researched symbols and put them together into a beautiful and unique piece of jewelry.

I lost it emotionally when he pointed out the sign of cancer engraved on the brooch. Strange as it may sound, it belonged there as a truly significant part of my life. On our return to Texas, the surprise continued. Jenn and Ashley flew home. Sarah had made a birthday video tape before she left for a year in Siberia, and she called to give personal greetings. Bob told me that he had arranged an "intimate" gathering for the evening, that turned out to be about sixty people. I got the usual gag gifts and funny cards about old age, but I told them all that I considered turning fifty to be a triumph since the alternative came too close when I was diagnosed with cancer.

As we approached the Christmas holiday, the poignancy of the second anniversary was less intense. In fact, I realized that I had forgotten the date of the mammogram, and I think that's good. On December 20, Jenn called to say "happy anniversary." I had to think for a minute since Bob's and my wedding anniversary was not until the next day. Then, I remembered what she meant. It seemed funny to hear "happy anniversary" for a day I remembered as so dreadful. But, Jenn reminded me that I could celebrate two years without a recurrence. That's a great way to look at it.

All three girls were home for Christmas, and it was just the five of us for a change. On Christmas morning, Bob surprised me again. The same Bangkok jeweler had make an 18-karat rose gold pin of the breast cancer ribbon. And, again, it made me cry. It told me that he clearly understood how profound this experience had been for me. After a wonderful day that even included some traditional Siberian customs introduced by Sarah, I received a special phone call from a young woman whom I had visited through Reach to Recovery. She had been having a very hard time, and she called to say that she did not want Christmas to pass without telling me how glad she felt to be alive and how thankful to have someone whom she did not even know before who cared enough to help, to visit and pray for her. Again, this brought lots of tears.

New Year's Eve brought another visitor, a very special role model whose spirit had encouraged me in my down times. Marilyn, suffering with multiple sclerosis, and her companion came from Austin to spend an afternoon with us. Decked out in her holiday gold tights, Marilyn slowly walked from the car to our door, using her walker. She was determined to get into the house on her own steam. What an inspiration. We held her standing between us for a photo, because this brave woman doesn't let anything get her down. She forced herself to stand and greet the new year with *joie de vivre*, encouraging all of us to do the same.

And With Thy Spirit

Susan Love said that a woman's life would never be the same again after losing a breast. I knew a few women with breast cancer who simply got back to business and forgot about cancer. Some of these women had escaped chemotherapy, and I wondered if that made a difference. Every morning when I awoke, I knew I was different. It was not traumatic to face my scarred, concave chest, but it was different and therefore reminded me that my life had changed. A friend wrote to me, after a visit we shared.

> *Something I didn't get around to asking you was whether you've had a spiritual awakening or a change of perspective or—I'm not even sure what words to use—but has your life changed in profound ways since you were diagnosed with cancer? You seem so calm. I wonder how you do it. You don't have to answer this soon (or ever), I was just wondering.*

I had not pondered that question deeply. I knew that I had achieved a real sense of calm during the period of the surgeries, and I attributed that to knowing clearly that I was receiving prayers from friends in many faiths. I also prayed differently than before. No longer were prayers pro forma, but I spent conscious time stating each name and exactly what I prayed for on behalf of each person. I would stop more often during the day and send out a quick prayer if I thought of someone in need. I had not become more "religious," per se, in terms of going to church or being born again. But I did feel as though life was different after cancer.

In asking the same question of me, another friend expressed real sadness that I had not had a born-again experience with the cancer journey. She encouraged me to invite Christ into my life. Her assumption that Christ was not already part of my life was incorrect. I believe that I was born a child of God. I was brought up a Christian, and my acceptance of other forms of worship simply makes me a better person, not less of a believer. Having not strayed from my beliefs, I did not feel the need to be born again.

After much thought, I responded:

> *I've spent more time than my silence would indicate thinking about your question of whether the cancer provoked any kind of spiritual experience. I'm still in the sorting out stage on that one and will let you know what I figure out. For one thing, I will tell you that I feel much less compulsive. I also feel much fuller knowing that who I am is important, as opposed to what I do. For me, that's fairly profound even though not religiously spiritual. I also feel very aware that this is a life-changing experience. Even though I may look the same to others, I don't feel the same.*

That belief created a dilemma. I did not feel the same, but I looked the same to others, creating confusion for those who had known me or had worked with me for a long time. Always an incredibly Type A personality, hard-charging, aggressive, competitive, ambitious, and motivated, I now found it difficult to motivate myself. I did not have to be in the front of the line every time, the most visible, the most recognized, the most out-spoken. For instance, the former Barbara would have continued working on the TRICARE challenge and become the spokesperson for every individual who contacted me. The new Barbara had made her statement, contributed to the new plan created by the process action team, and now wanted to back off and smell the roses.

I also found it difficult to break back into work. Leading a virtual company where the CEO resides miles away from the headquarters had never been easy for any of us at VIMA, and we continued to learn to make it work. However, during the many months of my treatment and recovery when my colleagues ran things smoothly without me, we all became accustomed to a different routine. I did not want to re-enter like a bull in a china shop, and without my daily presence, they often forgot to include me in business decisions. This dynamic, coupled with my own personal change in orientation, made it difficult to get on with things in a business sense.

A long e-mail conversation with Shannon helped us both as we tried to sort out what was going on for us spiritually and psychologically during the healing process. Neither of us had the answers, but the dialogue was helpful, insightful, and instructive. Shannon asked about my faith:

> *I know from your messages that you have faith. How did you come by it?*

Her question was helpful to me in my assessing the growth of my faith. I explained that I had been brought up an Episcopalian and was lucky to marry another Episcopalian. That made religious decisions easy for us. I was active as a child in Sunday school and youth group. I had gone to church camps for several summers. My hometown church was a center of my religious experience, where generations of my family had been baptized, confirmed, married, and buried.

I learned to pray from an early age, especially after my father passed away when I was eleven years old. The funeral home in our small town had been full when Daddy died, so we brought his body home before the funeral. Every night, I crept into the living room full of flowers, knelt by his coffin, and talked to God. After we had children, I said nightly prayers with our three girls, and I still prayed with Ashley when she was sixteen and the only child left at home. Sometimes my prayers were more like meditation. I would "talk" with God and feel a sense of calm. My nightly ritual now included The Lord's Prayer and then the name of everyone I knew who had cancer or another serious illness. I would ask God to give us all support, to keep our attitudes positive, to ease our pain, to help us into remission, and to prevent future recurrences.

Bob and I brought our girls up in the Church. Because we moved so frequently, we saw a lot of different parishes. Sometimes we were very active and liked the parish; other times we did not connect so closely. All the girls were confirmed, and they had been actively involved in church activities and youth groups at certain times of their lives. Our favorite church experience had been in California. When our family of five had gone to the Episcopal service on the first Sunday after Bob assumed command, we doubled the size of the congregation. Over the next year, we assumed many roles in the parish. The girls learned to acolyte. Sarah often played a hymn for the offering. Bob wrote outreach letters, inviting Episcopalians to join us at the unit chapel. Jenn started a Sunday school. Ashley baby-sat so parents could attend the service. The girls sponsored a Christmas pageant. I decorated the chapel. We felt like it was our very own parish.

I summarized that background for Shannon and remarked:

> *I don't talk much about my faith, and I don't use the expression that some people do when they say they "pray" about their problems or about decisions they need to make. It is very private to me, but it does give a sense of calm. Thanks for talking and listening to me. I hope we can continue to be a support to each other. I think of you every day and I do pray for your peace of mind through this long treatment.*

Shannon had her own struggles with denial, with emotional recovery, and with her faith. She aptly described the mix of emotions of cancer patients: grief, anger, depression, and a good deal of self-pity. I identified with her thinking that one day the doctors would call and say, "Whoops, made a mistake and we were looking at the wrong slides. You're really fine." Part of my emotional healing included coming to terms spiritually with the fact that I did have cancer, that no one made a mistake. It helped that I had received all my medical records, translated from French to English. Reading all the reports from the diagnosis through the surgeries, chemotherapy, and pathology findings helped make it all real. It was me, my own spirit and essence, that had cancer. My new spirit was that of a cancer survivor. My faith helped me through the process and would now help me find my way as a new person.

My search was similar to Shannon's, as she described herself:

> *I have to say that I'm in progress, in transition, as we all are, I guess. Sometime last year, in the throes of my treatment, and in the middle of many nights, I came to start to pray and to ask God for help, which I hadn't done in many, many years. And I started to find some comfort.*
>
> *Then, I felt a great deal of guilt that I only called on Him when I was in great need, and I didn't know what to do with all of those*

feelings. I am trying to listen to my heart and to what God is saying without judging or putting more demands on the whole process.

I ventured into church last week for the first time in about fifteen years. I went to give thanks to God for bringing me closer to Him over the last year or so. I was also very emotional about going back to church, which I feared that I would be. I was okay during the "talking" parts, but whenever the singing began, I started to cry. After the service, I was really crying, and I went out the back door.

I can't precisely say to you why I was so emotional, but it felt like overwhelming joy that God has brought me closer and closer, and some sadness that I have "erred and strayed like lost sheep." Practically, I'd like to go to church more regularly, but I can't go on sobbing in morning prayer amongst strangers. I believe that this will resolve itself, with God's help.

I clearly identified with Shannon's crying during the singing. When I thought back over the years, I remembered many instances of not making it through a hymn either because I was sad or very happy. I had never been able to make it through Silent Night on Christmas Eve, because I love the feeling of my family being together to celebrate Christ's birth.

When I thought about the times since my diagnosis when I had cried for joy, I thought more about nature and people. I had written months before about times when I simply caught my breath and held back the tears at the sheer joy of being alive, having survived the battle with cancer. Those tearful moments often happened when I watched one of the girls do something that made me so proud, when we were in the beauty of nature as on the mountain top in Utah, or when my family realized without my telling them that the cancer experience had made me a new person.

It is important to me to do things that nurture my spirit, a spirit created by and nurtured by a Superior Being. For me, that means spending time with people and in places where my being is happy and thoughtful. It means saying "no" to things that do not nurture my spirit. It means telling people how important they are to me and fighting for the things that will improve life for others. I believe that the new Barbara does not always cope as well under stress as the old Barbara. Fight or flight comes much more quickly than before. But, maybe I'm fooling myself and I never coped as well as I thought.

Afterword-And the Beat Goes On

As the journey continues, I am aware of having climbed over the wall that I hit head-on in December 1996. It felt like scratching and clawing for hand and footholds as I scaled the heights, but with incredible support from family and friends, with prayers and faith and hope, I came safely to the other side and life is richer, fuller, and more meaningful for having hit the wall.

Two years after my cancer treatment, I took time out to capture my journey on paper. The writing of this book served as a tremendous cathartic experience, but it certainly did not end the journey. At my two-year oncology appointment with Dr. Diehl, he said I could have a mini-celebration. The statistics for recurrence decline significantly for cancer patients who survive for two years. That sounded like good news. But, again, the good news often comes with the bad. He also explained that one is never out of the woods with breast cancer because it hides in the body. The five-year mark without recurrence, often considered so meaningful, is only another statistical event. Cancer patients may have recurrences of the original cancer long after the initial diagnosis.

After writing the book in Williamsburg, I returned to Texas and learned of the death of the woman who had led our Reach to Recovery group. Her recurrence had come quickly and aggressively. During my absence, my friends Mary Jane and Toni had both finished their stem cell transplants. Toni bounced back more quickly. Mary Jane continued to have problems with fevers and infections. A breast cancer support group was formed at the local Army hospital, sponsored by the American Cancer Society and the social worker at the hospital. I actively recruited new members and attended as often as possible. Support was important to me and it helped me to be a support to others.

As the spring approached, the American Cancer Society geared up for the annual Relay for Life. The people in Bob's command were incredibly involved, and together we formed four different teams to walk throughout the night and raise money for breast cancer. I was honored to be asked to give the opening remarks. Although asked to be upbeat and positive, I found it difficult to get through my prepared remarks without crying. So, I simply explained to the listeners that any tears expressed my emotion and conviction at how important their efforts were. I invoked the role models of Bea, Max, and Marilyn as I talked about the bravery of cancer patients. I talked about the value of support from friends and organizations like Reach to Recovery, sponsored by the American Cancer Society. I ended by saying:

> *We start this Relay for Life in hope, not in sadness. We are here for life, for help and hope for one another, and tonight we're here for fun as we share this experience together and join our forces to find a cure. Thank you for choosing life in your generous show of selflessness, camaraderie, and love for one another.*

Survivors walked the first two laps, and I linked arms with other survivors as we circled the track. The local newspaper had our photo on the front page of the paper on Saturday morning in our yellow survivor T-shirts. When the general relay began, Army units ran in step, parents with children in strollers ran or walked, little children eagerly kept up with parents, high school girls and Harley motorcycle riders, and old and young all walked for eighteen hours straight to raise money. It was an emotional experience to walk around the track and to see luminaries with my name on them.

Bob and I had placed fifty luminaries on the track along with hundreds of others that circled the entire quarter mile. They bore the names of our friends whom we honored as cancer survivors or victims. A wall of memory also included cut-out silhouettes with the same names. At 10 p.m., all the stadium lights were extinguished and only the luminaries lit the field while there was singing, poetry reading, and the roll call of all those honored as victims of the disease. It was truly moving. The next morning, my friend

Mary Jane closed the event with the promise "I'll be back" for the next year's Relay.

As spring turned to summer, I encountered more of what the doctors and cancer survivors had predicted. With minor medical problems, I continued to have frequent and sometimes painful tests to check for the possibility of uterine cancer and spread of breast cancer. I was grateful to find doctors who were concerned, willing to give me the tests, and accessible to me. Even after many biopsies, bone scans, x-rays, and blood tests, I find that I always have a real anxiety as I wait for test results. The fact that the original mammogram in 1996 came back with an answer I did not want means that I often fear that more tests will result in negative responses. And as I learned with the original diagnosis, it is the time of uncertainty waiting for test results that is the most difficult to bear.

Nonetheless, it is true that a new normalcy develops. In September 1999, Bob retired from the Army, and we left our friends in Texas to return to Virginia. That meant finding all new doctors, re-educating them about my case, establishing a new medical routine and a new support system. Reach to Recovery is not as active in northern Virginia, so I have made it my personal crusade to seek out breast cancer patients and support them through their treatment. I know firsthand that support can be by telephone and e-mail as well as face-to-face. During Breast Cancer Awareness month in 1999, I published an article on tips for survivors that was syndicated in newspapers across the country. I received several gratifying messages from readers that the information had helped them.

In January of 2000, Jenn challenged me to another incredible fundraiser. The Avon Breast Cancer Crusade was sponsoring a three-day, sixty-mile walk from Frederick, Maryland, to Washington, D.C. Jenn said that if I could beat cancer, I could walk for sixty miles. Having sold my interest in VIMA, I had time to train, and I spent months walking to prepare for several events. This became the season of walking in the Avon Three-Day, the American Cancer Society Relay for Life, and the Susan G. Komen National Race for the Cure. These experiences each added their own poignancy to the continuing journey of life as a breast cancer survivor.

As I trained, I pondered, "Why do we walk?" Each of the events involved walking or running in order to raise money to fight the disease, to find a cure, and to help underserved cancer patients to receive screening mammograms or treatment in the event of disease. Each event involved a team of supporters who contributed money or even walked together. Each involved a distance or amount of time that is more than a morning's stroll, thus requiring some effort.

Why do we walk for such a long time? Perhaps it is because the cancer experience lasts for a long time. One does not get over it in a few weeks or even months. With surgery, chemotherapy, and radiation, the treatment goes on and on and follow-up lasts forever.

Why do we walk for a long distance? It is because walking a long distance pushes us to limits we may be afraid that we cannot reach, a distance that feels too far and too frightening. A cancer diagnosis induces great fear. I had feared that I might lose my life, that I would not live to see my daughters grow up, not know my grandchildren. I feared pain and disfigurement. I feared that I would become a burden to others, that I would not be able to work, that I would lose my independence. The only way to overcome those fears and to go the distance was to persevere against what seemed insurmountable odds, to have faith that I could stay on track toward recovery. It was a long trek from ill to well, from victim to survivor, and I had to work hard to go the distance.

Why do we walk in teams or supported by teams? We walk with team support because one does not survive cancer alone. I thought of my medical providers, my family, and my e-mail support team that included people whom I had never met, friends of friends who had survived cancer and had good advice. I learned that, without a team around me, I was very depressed, and that I had to let that team help me in ways I could not even imagine. One does not survive cancer without the support of people on the team.

The Avon Breast Cancer three-day walk was an incredible challenge, taking a long time, going a long distance, and requiring a team effort. As the 2800 walkers passed schools, classrooms of children came out to cheer us on. Truck drivers beeped horns and waved. Business people and homeowners came to their doors to congratulate us. All along the route, friends and family erected signs and applauded us as we walked. And nearly 500 volunteers supported this three-day effort by setting up tent cities, serving three meals a day, providing snacks, water, porta-potties, and encouragement every couple of miles along the sixty-mile route. Jenn and I both admitted we could not have made the distance without one another.

The weekend was unseasonably hot and humid, and walkers dropped like flies, going to local hospitals for rehydration. Jenn and I managed to make the whole sixty miles by encouraging each other, putting ice in bandanas tied around our necks, and thinking of those friends with breast cancer whose names we wore on our shirts and hats. We were also inspired by an eighty-year-old Episcopal nun, herself a breast cancer survivor, who walked the whole route. The three-day walk concluded with a victory march along the Reflecting Pool to the Washington Monument. Survivors wore pink shirts and were cheered by our friends and fellow walkers as we entered the final staging area. It was incredibly emotional, inspirational, draining, grueling, and hot. But what a wonderful feeling of accomplishment.

During the spring, I also volunteered with the Susan G. Komen National Race for the Cure. At a media training session, I met an inspirational woman. Carolyn had advanced metastatic breast cancer. To look at her, she looked normal and healthy. She had her own short, blonde hair. She was cheerful and bubbly. She played a few holes of golf several times a week. But she cautioned us not to hug her or touch her with more than a gentle touch. Her bones were very fragile and she was often in pain.

Carolyn and I became e-mail buddies, and she was helpful to another friend of mine whose cancer returned to her bones. Carolyn had been married only for a short time, and she described her life as a willing of herself to live from one event to the next: her wedding, the birth of a niece, her high school reunion. Our e-mail acquaintance ended within a few months, when responses simply stopped coming. Despite my queries, I have not learned why, but I pray that Carolyn is free of pain. She will remain an inspiration to me.

When the National Race for the Cure was held in Washington, D.C., Rhonda came from Louisville and joined Bob, Jenn, Sarah, and me for the event. Along with 69,000 of our "friends," we walked through the streets of Washington, D.C., in the world's largest five-kilometer run/walk. Unable to join us, Ashley organized some of her sorority sisters to walk in the Newport News, Virginia, Race for the Cure. The family support was incredible.

My friends at the American Cancer Society in Texas invited me to return for their Relay for Life to give the closing speech. I enjoyed seeing friends from the Army, the community, and the American Cancer Society. But the return was both happy and sad. In giving the closing address a year earlier, my friend Mary Jane had promised, "I'll be back." What a joy to see her and to walk with her in the survivor's lap. But, Toni, who had undergone a stem cell transplant at the same time as Mary Jane, had died just one month earlier. I had felt devastated and helpless when I heard in January that Toni was hospitalized for metastasis to her brain. We had talked on the phone, and she showed the same indomitable spirit and faith in God that she always had. Throughout her ordeal, she was an inspiration, but she lived for less than three years from the time of her original diagnosis. I dedicated my remarks to Toni.

Toni personified why we walk. Her illness lasted a long time, three years. Her journey took her a long distance through every conceivable cancer treatment of slash/burn/poison and the realized fear that she would not see her son grow up. Toni belonged to a team, both accepting and giving support to others in need. As I closed my speech, with choking voice, I told them that I could hear Toni in her most positive voice, saying as she often did "Praise the Lord!" for the funds we had raised so that others would be saved from this disease.

In our season of walking, Jenn and I had raised nearly $20,000 to fight breast cancer. But the fight was far from over. In August, Mary Jane lost her battle. She fought to the end, as did Toni, with a positive attitude, with grace and dignity, and with a determination that she would contribute to the effort to find a cure.

There were clear lessons for cancer survivors in the lives of Toni, Mary Jane, and Carolyn. Survivorship means embracing the moment and living life to the fullest. It also means contributing to the future, to finding a cure so that our daughters will not suffer as we have. One must keep on walking with support and hope, while still contributing to a better life for others. Every day, over 500 women in the United States alone are diagnosed with breast cancer. Until we find a cure, the beat goes on.

Suggestions
for Survivors

Suggestions for Survivors

Even with early detection, a diagnosis of breast cancer is devastating news. How does one face a life-threatening illness with the positive attitude that has proven to help speed recovery and survival?

The diagnosis of breast cancer means addressing serious questions about treatment options. It also means taking action that allows you to focus on personal healing while home, family and career become secondary.

When I was diagnosed with breast cancer in 1996, I knew very little about the subject. I knew a handful of people who had survived, or died, from breast cancer. But the details escaped me. My doctor told me I had invasive ductal carcinoma. When I repeated that diagnosis to a specialist, I didn't even remember whether it was carcinoma or melanoma. Both are ugly words, and I didn't want either one.

The diagnosis made me feel inferior, flawed, and helpless. I felt incapable of functioning as a mother, wife, or business executive when I didn't even have control of my body. The months of treatment ahead seemed overwhelming until I began to take charge of my own attitude and my own care.

If you receive the same devastating diagnosis, don't hesitate—take charge. Being in charge puts you on the road to recovery. Here are some tips to help you face the road ahead.

Learn as much as you can about your type of breast cancer and the treatment options.

Soon after hearing of my diagnosis, I received *Dr. Susan Love's Breast Book*. It covers everything from A to Z about breast cancer and the options for treatment. It is written in a very readable style, taking the mystery out of the medical terminology that surrounds breast cancer.

Contact your local American Cancer Society. Get their brochures and ask for a visit by a Reach to Recovery volunteer. This volunteer is a breast cancer survivor. Along with an assortment of American Cancer Society reading materials, she will also bring you a temporary prosthesis if you had a mastectomy without reconstruction. If your doctor approves, she will show you arm and shoulder exercises that will help you recover strength and mobility in your arm and shoulder.

Interview your doctors and make your own decisions.

Depending on your diagnosis, you will have different decisions to make. My decisions were numerous. Could they get all the cancer with a lumpectomy or should they do a mastectomy, taking the whole breast? If I chose the mastectomy, did I want reconstruction or not? If I wanted reconstruction, would it be artificial implants or a flap of muscle from my stomach or shoulder? Did I need to have radiation, chemotherapy, pills, or a combination of these treatments?

All of these choices are very personal. Be informed and make the decision for your reasons, not what you think your doctor wants. You have the rest of your life to spend with yourself and your loved ones. Your doctors are important right now, but you will not be spending the rest of your life with them. Don't make hasty decisions. Take your time and consider your own lifestyle and future happiness, keeping in mind that no option is carefree. Look into the future maintenance requirements for each of the options you are facing

Build your own support group.

If a breast cancer support group is available, try it. I learned more about living with breast cancer from other survivors than from medical professionals. Survivors know about wigs, prostheses, and side effects of treatments. Survivors can explain what clothes will work if you have a mastectomy without reconstruction, or what future care is required if you have reconstruction. Equally important, survivors talk about how you feel as the months go on and you realize you must live as a breast cancer survivor with all the accompanying fears and hopes.

If there is no organized breast cancer support group available, build your own support group of family and friends. Talk to them about what is happening to you and how you feel. I formed an e-mail support group of over 100 people, some of whom I have never met. Friends of friends joined my e-mail group, many of them breast cancer survivors who helped me by telling their own experiences. Friends who lived far away were able to offer support, love, and prayers by communicating often over e-mail.

Tell people what you need.

Often friends would say to me, "Let me know what I can do for you." I felt uncomfortable telling them what I needed. I learned that it actually helped them feel better if they could help me. So, be prepared to tell your friends what you need: shopping, driving you to treatments, picking up your child from an activity, bringing a meal, or coming to walk with you or visit with you. Keep your list near the telephone so you are ready to say what it is that you need that day. If there is nothing specific you need, then assure your friends that the best thing they can do for you is pray for your recovery. Prayers are the most someone can do for you, not the least.

Spend time with people in pleasant places.

Although my doctor asked me to avoid crowds and places with children during the many weeks of chemotherapy treatments, I did not have to be alone. When I was alone too much, I felt very isolated and lonely. It is very important to be with others, to do "normal" things, and to be socially involved. Isolating yourself can cause depression which impedes healing. If you can't get out, then ask people to visit you. When my blood counts were very low, I wore a surgical mask. Friends won't mind wearing a mask if they can visit you and cheer you up.

When my counts were higher, my husband would take me on wonderful trips to old favorite places and exciting new places, making sure not to overdo. Despite the precautions, it gave us a happy time in the midst of battling the cancer.

Find reasons to laugh.

A positive attitude is a tremendous asset in healing. Friends supported my efforts at humor by sending e-mail jokes and funny stories, so I had several laughs a day. My e-mail support group held contests for the top ten reasons to have cancer or to be bald. My favorite response, from a bald male friend, was, "If you think your hair is more important than your brains, it probably is."

At home, my daughters and I watched old home movies together. We enjoyed great belly laughs as we watched the antics of the three girls when they were little.

If you are having chemotherapy, cut your hair first.

There is a big psychological advantage to cutting your hair rather than losing it down the drain. There are several practical reasons to cut your hair very short before having chemotherapy. First, losing your hair is very messy. It comes out over a period of days or weeks and gets on everything. Shower drains, pillow cases, and washing machines are full of hair. The shorter you cut it, the less mess.

Second, if you cut your hair off before it begins to fall out, then you are in charge. No one takes it from you. You decide when you lose it (up until about the first two weeks after your first chemotherapy session), so you feel as though you have beaten the "system."

Third, trying on wigs is a lot easier without a full head of hair. I bought a wig before I cut my hair off and tried to replicate my midlength style. What a disaster. I never wore the wig even after spending too much money on it. My success with wigs came when I ordered several synthetic wigs from a catalogue that allowed returns. I was able to try them on in the privacy of my own home and decide what would work best for me, then return the ones I didn't want. I found that the synthetic wigs looked absolutely natural and were totally carefree.

Exercise your affected arm and your whole body.

Daily exercise will help you have more energy even when treatments may drag you down. Continue any exercise regimen you did before cancer, or begin walking daily to get out and keep active. I found myself getting too lethargic when I didn't get out and walk.

Arm exercises are vitally important if you have a lymph node dissection. While it hurts to stretch those arm muscles and move that shoulder, the movement helps prevent more painful conditions later on, such as a frozen shoulder or swelling, called lymphedema. The American Cancer Society Reach to Recovery volunteers are trained to demonstrate particular arm and shoulder exercises that are beneficial for recovering full motion in your arm and shoulder. However, do not start the exercises until your doctor agrees you are ready.

Take stress out of your life.

This is a time to concentrate on getting well. Say "no" to all those non-essential tasks. For once in your life, put yourself first and be a bit selfish. Let a colleague take the business trip, or do it by teleconference. Ask someone who wants to help to bake those brownies for the school's bake sale, or just buy them. Do only those things that nurture your body and soul. You need to focus all your energy on healing. The healing process from a life-threatening disease is as much mental as physical.

Look at various work options. Consider working from home at your own pace. During periods of extended treatment and recovery, look at the possibility of going on disability. This was my choice, although I have many friends who have worked through periods of extended treatment. Consider what are your job demands and whether you are being fair to both yourself and your employer. You will not be as productive on the job during treatment. You will heal faster if you focus on yourself first.

Pamper yourself.

Let's face it, it is hard to feel beautiful with scars, a missing breast, radiation burns, or baldness. Spend time pampering yourself as often as possible. Get a weekly massage. Get regular manicures or pedicures. Go to a make-up specialist and learn how to change your make-up when you lose your eyelashes and eyebrows. The American Cancer Society's Look Good...Feel Better program offers free consultations.

If you don't have time, energy, or money for professional treatments, take long baths. Use nice bath oil or bubble bath and make yourself feel special. It is relaxing and invigorating, giving you more energy to focus on your own heeling.

Triumphing over breast cancer is a goal for all women and men who suffer from this disease. Our friends and families can support this goal by traversing this lonely path with us. Studies have shown that breast cancer patients with supportive families and friends do better in their treatment. Let's join together to triumph—and to find a cure for breast cancer.

Breast Cancer Organizations and Resources

Information and Counseling

AMC Cancer Research Center's Cancer Information and Counseling Line
Professional cancer counselors offer easy-to-understand answers to questions about cancer and will mail instructive free publications upon request. The service is equipped for deaf and hearing-impaired callers. Call Monday through Friday, 8:30 a.m. to 5:00 p.m., Mountain Standard Time.
Phone: (800) 525-3777

American Cancer Society
The American Cancer Society is the nationwide, community-based, voluntary health organization dedicated to eliminating cancer as a major health problem by preventing cancer, saving lives and diminishing suffering from cancer, through research, education, advocacy, and service. The toll-free hotline provides information on all forms of cancer and referrals to Reach to Recovery programs for breast cancer patients.
Phone: (800) ACS-2345
Web site: www.cancer.org

Breast Cancer Community
The Breast Cancer Community is an online community for information and support.
Web site: www.bclist.org

BreastCancer.Net Newsletter

The *BreastCancer.Net Newsletter* is delivered electronically free of charge to over 3,500 breast cancer survivors, health professionals, and legislators in fifty-four countries. Links to stories along with an archive of over 1500 other cancer-related news items are available twenty-four hours a day.

Web site: www.breastcancer.net

Breast Center

The Breast Center provides this resource for patients with metastatic breast cancer, Stage IV, or breast cancer recurrences.

Web site: www.patientcenters.com/breastcancer

Cancer Care Inc.

Cancer Care, Inc., is a social service agency providing support services, education and information, referrals, and financial assistance to cancer patients and their families.

Address: Cancer Care, Inc.
              275 7th Avenue
              New York, NY 10001
Phone: (800) 813-4673
Web site: www.cancercareinc.org
E-mail: info@cancercare.org

Cancer Information Service

The Cancer Information Service of The National Cancer Institute provides information and direction on all aspects of cancer through its regional network. It provides informational brochures without charge and refers callers to medical centers and clinical trial programs. Spanish speaking-staff members are available.

Phone: (800) 4-CANCER
Web-site: www.nci.nih.gov

CANSearch

CANSearch is a guide to cancer resources on the Internet compiled by the National Coalition for Cancer Survivorship.

Web site: www.cansearch.org

Gilda's Club

Gilda's Club provides places where people with cancer and their families can build social and emotional support.

Phone: (212) 686-9898

Web site: www.gildasclub.org

Mamm

Mamm Magazine provides a web site for women, cancer and community.

Web-site: www.mamm.com

National Lymphedema Network

National Lymphedema Network provides information on the prevention and management of lymphedema and supports research into the causes and possible alternative treatments for this condition.

Phone: (800) 541-3259

Web site: www.lymphnet.org

National Self-Help Clearinghouse

The National Self-Help Clearinghouse will refer callers to regional self-help services. Send a stamped, self-addressed envelope.

Address: National Self-Help Clearinghouse
               25 West 43rd Street, Room 620
               New York, NY 10036

Phone: (212) 354-8525

E-mail: gar@cunyvms1.gc.cuny.edu.

OncoLink

OncoLink is maintained by the University of Pennsylvania and provides resources on cancer and financial resources for patients.

Web site: http://cancer.med.upenn.edu

Planetree Health Library

Planetree Health Library is a nonprofit, consumer-oriented resource for health information. They prepare personalized packets of information, house a medical library that is open to the public, and offer information on both conventional medical as well as alternative treatments. Write or call for a catalog and price list.

Address: Planetree Health Library
                   2040 Webster Street
                   San Francisco, CA 94115
Phone: (415) 923-3680.

Wellness Community

The Wellness Community has extensive support and education programs that encourage emotional recovery and a feeling of wellness. All services are free. There are several locations around the country.

Address: Wellness Community
                   2716 Ocean Park Boulevard, Suite 1040
                   Santa Monica, CA 90405
Phone: (310) 314-2555
E-mail: TWCNATL@aol.com

Y-ME

Y-ME National Breast Cancer Organization provides breast cancer information, support and referrals through their national toll-free hotline. Trained volunteers, all of whom have had breast cancer, are matched by background and experience to callers whenever possible. Y-ME offers information on establishing local support programs and has eighteen chapters nationwide, in addition to their national headquarters in Chicago. Y-ME has also started a hotline for men whose partners have had breast cancer.

Address: Y-ME
                   212 W. Van Buren Street
                   Chicago, IL 60607
Phone: (800) 221-2141
                   (800) 986-9505—Spanish
Web site: www.y-me.org.

YWCA Encore Plus Program

The YWCA of the U.S.A.'s Encore Plus Program, located in member associations throughout the U.S.A., provides early detection outreach, education, post-diagnostic support, and exercise to all women. Call to find the location of the program nearest to you.

Phone: (800) 953-7567
                   (202) 628-3636

Advocacy and Fundraising

Avon Breast Cancer Crusade

The Avon Breast Cancer Crusade sponsors the Avon Breast Cancer three-day walks around the country, raising money for screening and treatment of underserved women and research to find a cure for breast cancer.

Web sites: www.avoncrusade.com

www.breastcancer3day.org

Susan G. Komen Foundation

The Susan G. Komen Foundation is a national organization with a network of volunteers working through local chapters and Race for the Cure® events across the country, funding education and screening projects in local communities for the medically underserved. Their mission is to eradicate breast cancer as a life-threatening disease by advancing research, education, screening, and treatment. Information on screening, breast self-exams, treatment, and support is available.

Address: The Susan G. Komen Breast Cancer Foundation

5005 LBJ Freeway, Suite 370

Dallas, TX 75244

Phone: (800) I'M AWARE

(800) 462-9273

(972) 855-1600

Web sites: www.breastcancerinfo.com

www.komen.org

www.raceforthecure.com

E-mail: helpline@komen.org

National Alliance of Breast Cancer Organizations

National Alliance of Breast Cancer Organizations (NABCO) is the leading nonprofit national resource for information and education about breast cancer. NABCO acts as an advocate for breast cancer patients and survivors in legislative and regulatory concerns.

Address: NABCO

9 East 37th Street, 10th Floor

New York, NY 10016

Phone: (888) 80-NABCO

                (212) 889-0606

Web site: www.nabco.org

National Breast Cancer Coalition

National Breast Cancer Coalition is a grassroots effort in the fight against breast cancer. It was formed in 1991 with the sole mission of eradicating breast cancer through action and advocacy.

Address: National Breast Cancer Coalition

              1707 L Street NW

              Suite 1060

              Washington, DC 20036

Phone: (202) 296-7477

Web site: www.natlbcc.org

The National Coalition For Cancer Survivorship

The National Coalition For Cancer Survivorship (NCCS) raises awareness of cancer survivorship through its publications, quarterly newsletter, education to eliminate the stigma of cancer, and advocacy for insurance, employment, and legal rights for people with cancer. NCCS also facilitates networking among cancer programs, serves as an information clearinghouse, and encourages the study of cancer survivorship. On a national level, NCCS provides public policy leadership on legislative, regulatory, and financing matters and promotes responsible advocacy among national cancer organizations.

Address: NCCS

              1010 Wayne Avenue, Suite 505

              Silver Spring, MD 20910

Phone: (301) 650-8868

                (888) 650-9127

Products and Cancer Supplies

The American Cancer Society's *Tlc catalogue* offers hats, turbans, scarves, sleep hats, and other products for cancer patients.
Phone: (800) 850-9445

Jodee After-Surgery Fashions offers mastectomy bras, prostheses, breast forms, and inserts.
Phone: (800) 821-2767

Paula Young Wigs offers a large variety of synthetic wigs.
Phone: (800) 343-9695

Recommended Books about Breast Cancer and Healing

Advanced Breast Cancer: A Guide to Living With Metastatic Disease (previously published as *Holding Tight, Letting Go*) by Musa Mayer (O'Reilly and Associates, 1998) includes treatment information and resources and is an excellent resource for patients and health professionals. It provides comprehensive information and resources covering many topics, including coping with the shock of recurrence, seeking information and making treatment decisions, communicating effectively with medical personnel, resolving family concerns, finding emotional and practical support, and handling disease progression and end-of-life issues.

A Helping Hand - The Resource Guide for People With Cancer (Cancer Care Inc., 1996). This handbook provides practical information about the kinds of help available to people with cancer and how to access these resources directly. Available free of charge by calling Cancer Care, Inc., (212) 221-3300.

A Woman's Decision: Breast Care, Treatment and Reconstruction by Karen Burger and John Bostwick (St. Martin's Press, 1998) offers readers information on breast cancer, treatment, and reconstruction. It covers every aspect of breast cancer from selecting a physician, to treatment, to how breast cancer affects relationships, to finding support groups and information on the Internet.

Be a Survivor: Your Guide to Breast Cancer Treatment by Vladimir Lange (Lange Productions, 1999) is informative, empowering, concise, and user-friendly. It is designed to help the patient and the family participate in the treatment and recovery. Developed in consultation with medical experts, it provides information about standard treatments, complementary therapies, and clinical trials.

Breast Cancer: The Complete Guide by Yashar Hirshaut and Peter Pressman (Bantam Doubleday Dell, 2000) is a thorough and accessible book on breast cancer with all the facts a patient needs to know.

Cancer as Initiation: Surviving the Fire by Barbara Stone (Open Court, 1994) describes the author's battle with cancer from a deep psychological and medical perspective. It includes dream analysis, the use of holistic healing methods, and Kirlian photography to track the cancer.

Cancer Survivor's Club: A Nurse's Experience (previously published as *Joining the Club*) by Lillie Shockney (Windsor House, 1997) describes the author's experience with breast cancer. It includes advice from a nurse's perspective on how to talk to your doctor and your family and provides intimate details about a woman's femininity following mastectomy.

Cancer Talk by Selma Schimmel and Barry Fox (Broadway Books, 1999) is a collection of the voices of cancer survivors, nurses, doctors, social workers, family, and friends of cancer patients. It comes from "The Group Room," a call-in radio show that grew to be the world's largest cancer support group.

Dr. Susan Love's Breast Book by Susan M. Love, M.D. (Addison Wesley, 1995) is the bible of books on breast physiology, including cancer and potential treatments. It is written by a physician about her observations of patient experiences and includes extensive medical information.

I'm Alive and the Doctor's Dead by Sue Buchanan (Zondervan Publishing, 1998) is a high-spirited story for any woman facing a medical verdict she does not want to hear. It assures women that there is life during and after cancer.

It's Always Something by Gilda Radner (Avon, 1995) is an autobiographical account of the famous comedienne and actress which ends with her three-year battle against ovarian cancer.

Living Beyond Breast Cancer by Marissa Weiss, M.D. and Ellen Weiss (Times Books, 1998) prepares the breast cancer patient for any eventuality as treatment ends and the rest of life begins.

Love, Medicine and Miracles by Bernie S. Siegel, M.D. (Harper Perennial, 1990) describes how love heals. Miracles happen to exceptional patients every day, patients who have the courage to work with their doctors to participate in and influence their own recovery.

My Breast by Joyce Wadler (Pocket Books, 1997) describes the author's experience with breast cancer as a single, career woman. She describes taking control of her choices for treatment and the relationships with family, friends, and lovers during this time.

My Mother's Breast: Daughters Face Their Mothers' Cancer by Laurie Tarkan (Taylor Publishers, 1999) offers support for the loved ones of breast cancer patients. It contains touching stories of sixteen daughters of all ages who must deal with the pain and devastation of their mothers' illness. It brings to light the unique emotional issues daughters face, including the fears for their own health.

Not Now—I'm Having a No Hair Day by Christine Clifford (Pfeiffer Hamilton, 1996) a humorous book filled with cartoons, describes the author's treatment for breast cancer and the use of humor for healing.

Quantum Healing by Deepak Chopra (Bantam Books, 1990) is a book filled with the mystery, wonder and hope of people who have experienced seemingly miraculous recoveries from cancer and other serious illnesses.

Spontaneous Healing by Andrew Weil, M.D. (Fawcett Columbine, 1995) presents medical knowledge from around the world to explain the human healing system.

The First Year of the Rest of Your Life: Reflections for Survivors of Breast Cancer by Nancy Brinker and Charla Hudson Honea (Pilgrim Press, 1997) is a collection of stories and reflections of women who have had breast cancer and their desires to save others from the same disease.

The Healing Journey: Overcoming the Crisis of Cancer by Alastair J. Cunningham (Key Porter Books, 1992) is written by a scientist to help cancer patients and their families in making rational decisions between the conservatism of Western medicine and the radicalism of New Age healing.

The Race is Run One Step at a Time by Nancy Brinker and Catherine McEvilly Harris (Summit Publishing, 1995) tells about the author's sister, Susan G. Komen, and the author's experiences with cancer which led to the founding of the Susan G. Komen Breast Cancer Foundation. It provides a guide to medical care, which is becoming somewhat outdated.

The Red Devil by Katherine Russell Rich (Three Rivers Press, 2000) tells the intimate story of a young career woman diagnosed with breast cancer who suffers a debilitating recurrence and survives through far-reaching treatment.

Woman to Woman: A Handbook for Women Newly Diagnosed With Breast Cancer by Hester H. Schnipper and Joan Feinberg Berns (Wholecare, 1999) is a book in which survivors of breast cancer offer warm, practical advice, essential information, and reassurance to newly diagnosed women.

Where the Buffaloes Roam: Building a Team for Life's Challenges by Bob Stone and Jenny Stone Humphries (Addison Wesley, 1993) describes Bob Stone's battle with cancer and the support he received by putting together a team of family and friends to help him through the hard times of treatment and recovery.

Barbara Pate Glacel Ph.D

Barbara Pate Glacel has followed the course of diverse and challenging careers over the last three decades.

As a human relations professional, Dr. Glacel began her career in academia, teaching business and political science at several educational institutions, including the University of Alaska and Central Michigan University. In 1984, she moved into the private sector, working in management first for ARCO Alaska and then for the Hay Group, and finally founding her own company, VIMA International—The Leadership Group, where she acted as CEO for twelve years. Having sold her interest in VIMA, Dr. Glacel continues to serve a select number of clients in executive coaching, team development, and organizational change. She has authored three books and numerous articles, and is a frequent public speaker.

Married for thirty-one years to career Army officer Brigadier General (Retired) Robert Glacel, Barbara is the mother of three grown daughters: Jennifer, Sarah, and Ashley. In addition to maintaining a household and raising a family while moving often, as dictated by the needs of the military, she also became involved in a number of Army policy issues. She actively volunteered in the many Army communities in which she lived and was appointed to several committees, including the Department of Defense Science Board Quality of Life panel in 1995 and the Army Science Board from 1986 to 1990. She currently serves on the prestigious Defense Advisory Committee on Women in the Services, whose civilian members were selected for their achievements in their professions and civic affairs.

As a breast cancer survivor since 1997, Barbara has become an advocate for others facing this disease, working to provide early detection as well as to find a cure. Through the American Cancer Society Reach to Recovery program, she volunteers her time advising breast cancer patients. She has walked hundreds of miles in the American Cancer Society Relays for Life, the Susan G. Komen Foundation Races for the Cure, and the Avon Breast Cancer 3-Day sixty-mile walks, fundraising many thousands of dollars through her efforts. She also testified before the Subcommittee on the Civil Service of the United States House of Representatives Committee on Government Reform and Oversight about the need for improved access to medical care in the military. She speaks and writes about cancer and survivorship nationally and overseas.

Living each day as a breast cancer survivor, Barbara enjoys her family, her friends, and meaningful work with a new perspective on life. She welcomes readers to contact her at BPGlacel@aol.com

Order Form

Qty.	Title	Price	Total
	Hitting the Wall	$16.95	
	Shipping and handling Add $3.50 for orders under $20, add $4.00 for orders over $20		
	Sales tax (WA residents only, add 8.6%.)		
	Total enclosed		

Telephone orders:
Call 1-800-461-1931
Have your Visa or
Mastercard ready.

E–Mail orders:
E–mail your order request
to harapub@foxinternet.net

**International
Telephone orders:**
Toll free 1-877-250-5500
Have your credit card ready.

Fax orders:
Fax completed order form to
(425) 398-1380.

Postal orders:
Send completed order form to:
Hara Publishing
P.O. Box 19732
Seattle, WA 98109.

Payment: Please check one
☐ Check
☐ Visa
☐ MasterCard

Name on Card: _____

Card #: _____

Expiration Date: _____

Name _____

Address _____

City _____ State _____ Zip _____

Daytime Phone (_____) _____

Quantity discounts are available. Call (425) 398-2780 for more information.

Thank you for your order!